INTERMITTENT FASTING OVER 50

The Ultimate and Complete Guide for Healthy Weight Loss, Burn Fat, Slow Aging, Detox Your Body and Support Your Hormones with the Process of Metabolic Autophagy

Amanda K. Loss

- Table of Contents -

Introduction

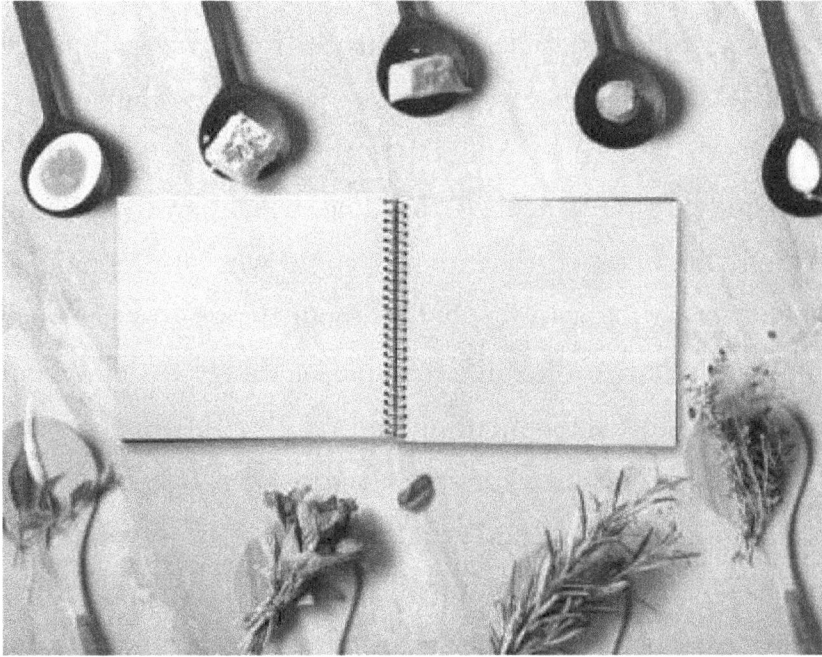

Thank you so much for purchasing *Intermittent Fasting Over 50: The Ultimate and Complete Guide for Healthy Weight Loss, Burn Fat, Slow Aging, Detox Your Body, and Support Your Hormones with the Process of Metabolic Autophagy.* In this book, we will talk about intermittent fasting, and more specifically on how someone should follow intermittent fasting if they are above the age of 50.

Many people don't realize it, but intermittent fasting is fantastic for people who are above the age of 50 as it helps them to slow down aging and detoxify their bodies. One of the main things to worry about once you get up to the age of 50, is that you need to heal the body the right way so that you can slow down the aging process. Who doesn't want to live for a very long time and be healthy at the same time? Everybody wants to achieve this goal, which is why we have written this book so that many people who are looking to slow down aging or to feel better about themselves can read along and change their life. Couple of things to remember before you start implementing and reading this book; make sure that you consult with your doctor before you begin any plan. The truth is we don't know what situation you are in, which is why we recommend that you consult with a professional before you start intermittent fasting as it cannot be ideal for everyone. Another thing to remember would be that intermittent fasting has to be done correctly; so make sure that you understand everything in this book before you start implementing the tips and tricks. Other than that, you should be good to go when it comes to intermittent fasting.

Chapter 1: What Is Intermittent Fasting?

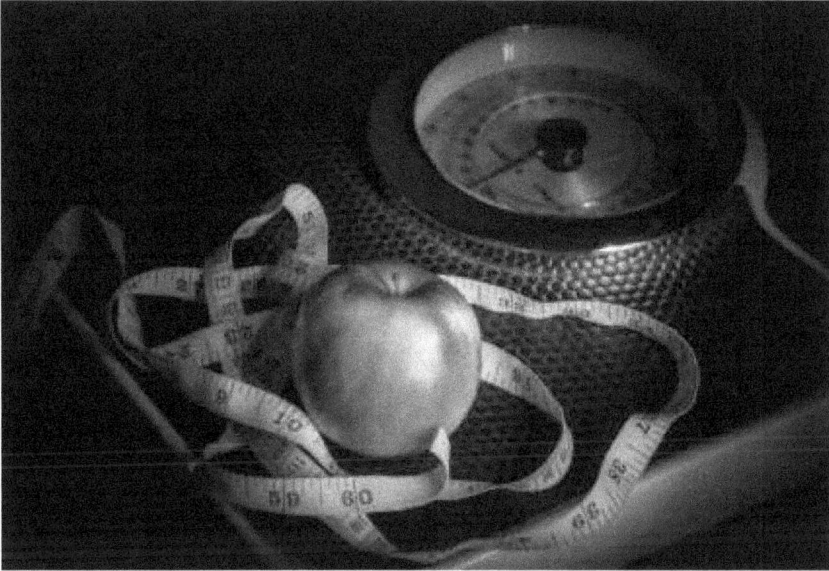

In this chapter, we will talk about intermittent fasting, and what it means to follow intermittent fasting. If you have been living under a rock, there's a high chance that you have no idea what intermittent fasting is or what it can do for you. What we will do is go through the basics of intermittent fasting so that you understand what intermittent fasting is, and that you have a better understanding of it moving on. A quick disclaimer; this chapter might be boring to many people as the information is very remedial. However, this information to some might be new, so if you find this chapter boring, then you are free to skip it. However, if you're still iffy about intermittent fasting or that you have no idea exactly what it does, then we recommend that you stick around. Time and time again, people have followed different types of fad diets, which may or may not work for them. Even if they do work for them, chances are they would give up very quickly and gain back the weight or the results that they achieved. The reason why they would give up and go back to the normal cell is that it is straightforward not to make it a habit or to make it a lifestyle.

The problem with modern-day and fad diets is that it is simply not sustainable in the long-term. If you want to lose weight and feel better by yourself for the rest of your life, then you need to pick something which is not only sustainable but can be adjusted into your lifestyle based on your needs. Moreover, you need something that gives you the freedom to eat and have whatever it is that you like in moderation so that you can enjoy life and be with your friends and family a lot more often. The truth is, many fad diets do not allow you to eat food, which is unhealthy. Don't get me wrong; eating unhealthy food all the time is not the best thing for your body anyway.

However, we recommend that you eat decent quality food often, so that you see the benefits that you are looking for when it comes to losing fat or building muscle. However, eating decent food all the time can be a tedious task, which can lead to failure in the long-term, which is why having unhealthy food, which tastes good here and there can lead to overall success in the long-term. With that being said, following fat diets play does not allow you to eat anything that is unhealthy. Most of the time, the fad diets put you in a position where you are insanely starving your body. Starving your body in the short-term might lead to weight loss, which might make you feel better; however starving yourself in the long-term can lead to many unwanted health fallbacks.

This is another reason why people who start following fad diets tend to give up so soon. This is where intermittent fasting comes in; the great thing about intermittent fasting is that many people don't even switch up what they are eating. What they do is eat cyclically. They would eat for certain hours of the day and would not eat for certain hours of the day. In essence, intermittent fasting is a cyclical way of eating. Now the most common way for people to follow intermittent fasting would be the 16/8 method. And this method you will be eating for 8 hours of the day, and you will be fasting for 16 hours of the day.

This is where you will not get any food to eat, and we'll have to survive on water or black coffee. You can have anything you want, which has no calories when you are fasting. Now there are tons of intermittent fasting methods, which we will talk about later on in this book. However, the 16/8 method has been working very well for most people and can be added to their lifestyle. The great thing about this method would be that you don't have to worry about having certain hours to be more important than others when it comes to eating window and vice-versa. You will be the one picking out the times for your eating window and your fasting window. The most common times for fasting are 8 pm till 12 pm the next day, then eating from 12 pm to 8 pm, again this time could be whatever works for your schedule.

Another great thing about intermittent fasting would be that there are no restrictions on what you could be eating. For example, during the eating window, many people eat whatever they want within reason to achieve their goals. I have seen many Fitness professionals eat food such as buttermilk biscuit, or even candy and dessert sometimes during the eating window, and still lose weight. We don't recommend you do that. However, this plan gives you the freedom to eat whatever you want while still seeing the results when it comes to losing fat and building muscle.

If you want to lose fat even more efficiently with intermittent fasting, we recommend that you eat a good, well-balanced diet slightly in a caloric deficit. This will allow you to not only lose fat but also to be certain that you're going to see results in the long-term when it comes to overall health and well-being. We also recommend that you accompany this with a fitness plan, make sure that you're working out in the gym if you want to lose fat and see the results that you have been hoping for. Another great thing about intermittent fasting, especially for people who are over the age of 50 years, is that it slows aging. One of the very best things, when it comes to intermittent fasting would be that it allows you to have very well-balanced aging and makes you look younger. These are thanks to two things, and the first one would be the increase in growth hormone. As you may know, intermittent fasting has shown to increase growth hormone production. This hormone is the youth of foundation; the reason why is because it will help you to recover quickly.

The benefits of growth hormone also include better skin and better bones, and you will also lose more fat and build more muscle. Another thing that intermittent fasting helps with would be the process known as autophagy. Autophagy is a process where your body gets rid of old/dead cells and replaces them with new cells.

This is the reason why you see the youth benefits, and the reason why many people stay young for a very long time.

These detoxifying cells would also mean getting rid of any diseased cells, which may include cancerous cells. Many people claim to get rid of their cancer very quickly by following intermittent fasting, and we can't back that up; however, it has been claimed by many cancer survivors. If you're someone looking to not only be better when it comes to Performance inside and outside the gym, but also to look a lot younger in the long-term, then you have no reason not to follow intermittent fasting. We will make it very easy for you when it comes to picking out the right plan and how to follow it appropriately.

Understand this, and intermittent fasting could be one of the easiest plans you could follow. And it all starts by reading this book. Have you already taken the first step to seeing better results with your body and health? Make sure that you go all the way with it. Intermittent fasting is like eating in increments. As we told you, it is a cyclical way of eating food, which allows you to consume all the calories you need in a certain hour of the day, while in certain time of the day, you will be fasting and not eating anything at all. Once you start following intermittent fasting, you will be surprised how much time we spend on eating food. We spend a lot of time, more specifically waste a lot of time eating food. If you're someone who is looking to see success with their business or their work environment, then you will gain from that time and see the results that you have been hoping for. Intermittent fasting truly is a win-win situation. It makes you feel younger, and it gets rid of any bad cells in your body, while increasing all the good hormones. Think of it this way, and there are many people who follow intermittent fasting without even knowing it. Many religions recommend that you fast for 30 days, or however long. This goes to show intermittent fasting has been in practice for a very long time, and good reason, it simply works.

Now, if you are someone who can't fast every day for the rest of your life, don't worry as you will have at least one day in the week or you can eat throughout the whole day. We recommend that you do that as it will allow you to be more motivated in the long-term, which is what intermittent fasting is all about; it is about creating a lifestyle. If you are tired of following diets that yield you some results, but they aren't sustainable in the long-term, then chances are intermittent fasting is going to be your savior.

Make sure that you pick the plan that fits your needs and your goals. We will talk about all the intermittent fasting methods later on in this book. However, once you understand the benefits and the reasons why you need to be following intermittent fasting, then it will be straightforward for you to follow it in the long-term. The main thing that differentiates intermittent fasting to any other fad diet is that the health benefits of intermittent fasting, and not just aesthetic benefits. Meaning, God guides and gives you a set of promises which may or may not be delivered. However, intermittent fasting has shown time and time again to deliver aesthetic benefits, and on top of that, help you get rid of many diseases that will help you stay healthy for a very long time.

Intermittent fasting is also one of the best plans to follow up for someone who's over the age of 50. The reason why we say so you is because it helps you to stay younger and to enjoy life a lot more. When you're 50, the main thing you want to do is enjoy life, and if you want to enjoy life, then you need to be in a healthy State of Mind and Body. Intermittent fasting gives you all of that, and on top of that, it helps you to stay a lot younger for a very long time. If you don't believe me, then look at your celebrities; many celebrities who are in their 50s tend to follow intermittent fasting and for an excellent reason. It is because it helps them to stay younger and to think a lot better and quickly.

Finally, intermittent fasting helps you to save a lot more time because you will not be thinking about eating for a certain amount of time, which will allow you to spend that time working on your craft. With that being said, we now conclude this chapter. The main take-home message from this chapter would be that intermittent fasting can be used for numerous reasons, if you are someone looking to gain muscle or lose fat or you want to be younger for a long time. In addition, intermittent fasting is something that should be considered more of a lifestyle than something that is to be done once every two months. Now, if you are serious about changing your life, and about starting living healthier, then intermittent fasting is the answer for you.

Chapter 2: Benefits of Intermittent Fasting

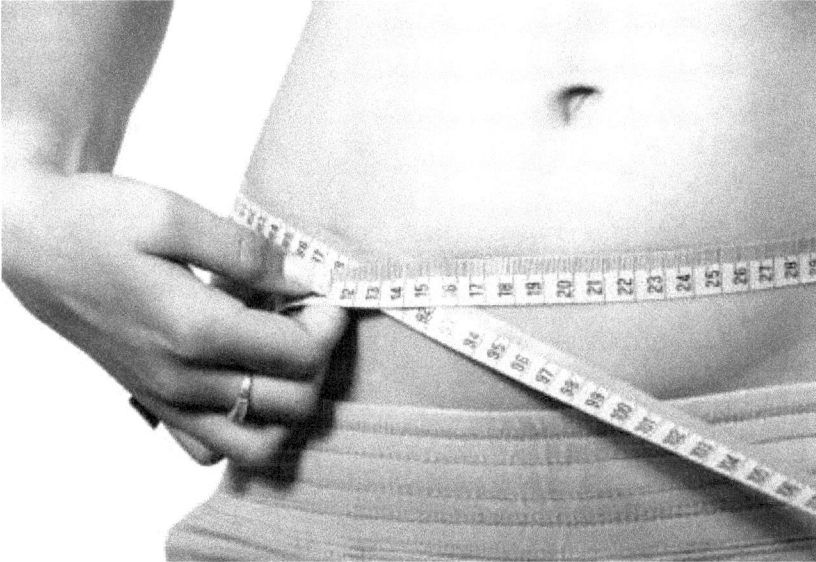

Now that you have a clear idea of what intermittent fasting is, let's talk about some of the benefits that come along with intermittent fasting. The truth is many benefits come along with intermittent fasting, and they have all of them backed up by science. Keeping that in mind, we will now talk about some of the significant benefits which come along with intermittent fasting so that you can get a better idea of why you should follow it and how it can be beneficial to you. One thing to remember is that all these benefits are great, but you must make sure that you are fit to follow intermittent fasting if you're not fit and healthy to support intermittent fasting than we would advise you not to follow it. The best way to find out if you can observe intermittent fasting is to consult with your doctor before you do any such plans, enough of that let's get into the topic of benefits.

Weight loss

As you know, intermittent fasting has been shown time and time again to help people lose body fat, and the keyword is body fat, as many people consider weight loss to be the key. If you're losing muscle, then there's no benefit of losing weight, as losing muscle can cause many health hazards. On the other hand, if you're losing body fat, then it could be perfect for you as it can lower the risk of many other diseases that come along. Many people who start falling intermittent fasting notice a decrease in body fat, and the reason why that is is that you are not spiking your insulin all the time and converting all those carbs into fat.

As you know, when you eat anything, your insulin goes up, and if it does not have time to use up all those calories in glycogen, it will be stored into fat. The great thing about intermittent fasting is that you don't have to worry about getting all those glycogens stored into fat as you will not be eating so frequently. When you're not eating so often, then you will start burning body fat that you already have. They're for preserving your muscles while using body fat for the energy source. The great thing about that is, you will not be using any glycogen at all and merely be burning off that excess body fat. You see, when you're intermittent fasting, your body goes into starvation mode, which is healthy for you. We have evolved to live without food for a couple of days, so it is our natural habitat not to eat food all the time. What intermittent fasting does helps us with our back in the daily routine and use body fat for energy?

Muscle gain

There have been many studies showing that intermittent fasting can help you put on muscle, and the truth is that intermittent fasting is perfect for putting on muscle and losing body fat. When you're intermittent fasting, your body will be increasing your hormone production of growth hormone and testosterone. Especially in men, which is why intermittent fasting is the ideal scenario for natural athletes to put on muscle. If you're someone who's abusing steroids, then there's no benefit for you to use intermittent fasting when it comes to putting on muscle. However, if you use the healthy route and not use any steroids, then intermittent fasting can be the answer for you. When you're intermittent fasting, your growth hormone can go up to 4000% office natural levels.

As you know, growth hormone has been shown to put on and preserve muscle while increasing your bone density. This is a no-brainer for natural athletes, as you will be increasing your testosterone and growth hormone at the same time you will put on muscle. On the other hand, you will also be cleaning out your gut, which will help you digest food a lot more efficiently. Many people don't know this. Still, intermittent fasting can help you clean out your stomach, having a healthy gut is very important when you're looking towards putting on muscle so make sure that you consider that when starting any muscle gaining plan.

Mental fog.

Intermittent fasting has also been shown to reduce mental fog. As you know, mental fog can be one of the most annoying things you can face when you're trying to achieve something in your work or personal life. What intermittent fasting does is help you not worry about digesting and focus on feeding your brain. Let me explain when you're eating all the time your body concentrated on understanding the food. When you're intermittent fasting body does not have to worry about food and in fact, give you the mental focus you need. Most of the time, people cannot focus on is because they don't have the energy to concentrate as their body is digesting their food. As simple as a sound, but it's true when you're not understanding, you are a lot more focused on the work that you're doing only because your body has nothing else to do. If your organization is free of any digestion on any other thing that it has to focus on, that's when you can take up all the things you want to do, so if you're going to focus a lot more and rid of the mental fog, your body will facilitate that for you very directly. Also, there have been many scientific studies showing that intermittent fasting, along with ketogenic diet, can help you tremendously to focus. As you know, insulin production can help us feel a lot more lethargic, which is why when following a ketogenic diet and intermittent fasting, insulin levels won't be out of whack. Therefore, you will have a lot less mental fog and a lot more mental clarity and focus.

Reduce blood pressure:

As you know, intermittent fasting as shown to reduce blood pressure, which makes it an excellent plan for people to follow when it comes to putting on muscle and losing body fat. If you're eating a lot more food, which should be our goal when it comes to putting on muscle, then chances are your blood pressure will be going up. However, when you're following intermittent fasting, that's something you don't have to worry about it, like intermittent fasting, as shown to reduce blood pressure. There have been many scientific studies showing that intermittent fasting can and will lower blood pressure. So it is one of the best things to follow when it comes to lowering your blood pressure and to see better health benefits overall. Whether it is your goal to lose fat or build muscle having a lower blood pressure is very crucial for you as well help your cardiovascular health and wellness. Cardiovascular health and wellness are essential as a house you live a long, fruitful life, so keep that into consideration when following intermittent fasting.

Lower cholesterol levels

Recently there was a 3-week study showing that intermittent fasting can reduce cholesterol levels tremendously. In the study, it showed that people reduce their bad cholesterol by a couple of points. Without getting to sign to pick on you, intermittent fasting has been scientifically proven to lower the bad cholesterol in your body. If you are facing cholesterol issues, then definitely consider intermittent fasting as a can help you with lowering cholesterol levels. Cholesterol is a silent killer in the United States, which is why it is essential to understand how cholesterol works and how it can help you or hinder you. Meaning the right amount of natural cholesterol level is critical, however when it gets too high, and it is mostly the wrong cholesterol level, then the chances are that you are not in the right place when it comes to health. Which is why it is essential to understand how cholesterol levels work and how to reduce them, if you're following intermittent fasting then that's something you don't have to worry about as it does everything for you.

Cancer

Intermittent fasting is also shown to reduce the risk of cancer. As you know, cancer grows in our body very rapidly. There have been many scientific studies showing that intermittent fasting can help us get rid of cancer once and for all. If you didn't know, there was one man who fasted for ten days Non-Stop and got rid of his disease. We don't know how accurate that is, and please don't put us on it, but this is what people have been saying about intermittent fasting and cancer. Intermittent fasting is indeed the new way to get rid of cancer, as much professional say. Having to control what you eat and when you eat it is essential, what intermittent fasting does is that it allows us to get rid of all the bad cells in our body by using a full cycle known as autophagy. General Autophagy as a process where your body gets rid of the old battery and makes new cells in your body. This is why intermittent fasting can and will reduce the risk of cancer, consider that when following intermittent fasting.

Reduce insulin resistance

As you know, intermittent fasting can reduce insulin sensitivity, which is why intermittent fasting has to be followed by many people if they want to see better results. Insulin sensitivity is significant, and being insulin resistant means that you will not be digesting any food that is going into your body. Many people who have diabetes tend to be insulin resistant, controlling this hormone is very important for overall health and longevity. What intermittent fasting does as it does not spike up your insulin randomly, what it gives you as a leveled insulin level product that will help you not only to say healthy but to help you digest food. This is very important when you're following intermittent fasting and trying to live a long healthy life; controlling this hormone wall dictates how well and how many diseases you can avoid in the future. Make sure you use intermittent fasting for the right reasons, meaning taking care of your health and body. There have been many scientific studies showing that intermittent fasting will make you a lot more insulin sensitive, which is something we want as we get older; we become more insulin resistant.

Increase longevity

With all these benefits comes durability, we have been talking about it briefly in this chapter so far. But as you can see, intermittent fasting and definitely help you with longevity and how long you will live. Which is why periodic fasting is one of the most basic eating plans to follow when it comes to overall health and wellness, the truth is that intermittent fasting will not only help you put on muscle and lose body fat, but it will help you to live a longer life overall. Understanding this is very important when it comes to bettering your life, you have to realize that health is not just about looking good and feeling good it is about longevity and how long you stay healthy for. What intermittent fasting provides you with, is the reduction of any diseases, or attracting any conditions and on top of that, giving you the health and body that you want. Intermittent fasting can indeed increase your longevity. In combination with all these benefits, intermittent fasting can genuinely help you understand what life is about. Increase longevity will give you a lot more benefits such as you get older, and you will not have any health complications or minimal; on top of that, you will not be taking any medications or needing any if you follow a healthful eating plan like intermittent fasting.

DNA

Intermittent fasting has been shown to preserve your DNA and to keep it healthy, and we will not get into this topic to genuinely as it has not been backed up by science as much. However, there have been many studies showing that intermittent fasting will help you not only to fight off any hazardous issues with your DNA, but it will help you preserve it. Preserving your DNA is very important, which is why you need to follow intermittent fasting.

Fertility

Intermittent fasting has been shown to increase productivity in men, as the hormone production goes up, so does the fertility. If you are a man looking to improve your sperm count, then there is no better way for you to go about it than to follow intermittent fasting. This will naturally increase your fertility without messing with any medications, and it is always best for you to increase your sperm count through natural means than to take any medications for it, definitely consider intermittent fasting when trying to increase sperm count or to increase fertility. Now there have been some things that intermittent fasting can increase women's fertility as well. However, we will not tell you that it does, for sure, as it has not been backed up yet.

Cell rejuvenation

As you know, intermittent fasting has been very well-known for autophagy, which is a cell rejuvenation process. When it comes to intermittent fasting and cell Rejuvenation, they going hand-in-hand. If you're looking to better your health and detoxify your body fully, then there's no better way to go about it later to follow intermittent fasting. Make sure that you follow intermittent fasting for the right reasons, which means that you're trying to detoxify your body inside and out. Intermittent fasting will not only detoxify your gut, but it will also detoxify yourself the way it functions everything that you can think of intermittent fasting while detoxified. The truth is that, most of the time, humans are spending their time digesting their food. Therefore, they get in no time to detoxify themselves. We need to detoxify your body naturally, and that comes through starvation, which is why intermittent fasting is one of the best ways to not only rejuvenate yourself but to detoxify your body.

Detox

Now that we have extensively talked about cell rejuvenation let's talk about detoxification and how it works and intermittent fasting. When you're fasting, your body does not have to worry about digestion, which is why it is an excellent idea for your body to start detoxifying itself. This is one of the reasons why he will feel a lot cleaner internally when following intermittent fasting. Many people who follow intermittent fasting feel completely detox within 15 days of starting the plan.

Moreover, intermittent fasting will Detox by everything in your body that you can think about, from your nails to your hair to every single cell in your body. Intermittent fasting is a lot more thorough than a green drink detox, which is why periodic fasting is highly recommended by not only fitness experts but doctors these days. Detoxifying your body is significant, and it is similar to getting an oil change in your car. If you want to keep your vehicle nice and to run, then you need to do regular maintenance, which includes oil change, the same thing goes with your body, which is why you need to detoxify your body as often and as thorough as you can.

Reduce stress and inflammation

Intermittent fasting has shown a significant reduction in inflammation. As you know, information causes a lot of many chronic diseases such as Alzheimer's, dementia, obesity, diabetes, and much more. Now, there are many ways that intermittent fasting helps you get rid of inflammation. The first one being autophagy, as you know, intermittent fasting helps you with cell rejuvenation cleans up itself by eating out the old self and rejuvenating them with the newer, stronger ones. If your body does not rejuvenate itself with more new cells, the older ones that have stayed for an extended period can cause inflammation.

As you know, the average diet does not allow for cell rejuvenation to happen; this is where intermittent fasting comes in as it has been proven to help with the process of autophagy. Another way intermittent fasting enables you to get rid of inflammation would be by producing ketones. When you are fasting, your body uses up all the glycogen stores, which makes it start using stored fat for fuel, and when fats are broken down for energy, ketones are produced. One of the most popular ketones in your body will block a part of your immune system, which is responsible for inflammatory disorders. Another way intermittent fasting helps you lower the risk of inflammation is by making you insulin sensitive. When your body becomes insulin resistant, you will be holding much glucose in your bloodstream. More glucose in your blood will create inflammation, and intermittent fasting allows your body to get rid of all the glucose, which helps you reduce inflammation in your body.

Now that we've talked about many ways intermittent fasting enables you to reduce inflammation, let's talk about how intermittent fasting can help you get rid of stress. You see, inflammation and stress go hand in hand. If you have high levels of inflammation, chances are your stress levels are going to be higher. This means that if you lower your inflammation, you will reduce your stress levels, and as you know, fasting helps with better brain function. Intermittent fasting enables you to send better signals to your brain, which would equal a better functioning brain.

When your mind is functioning at its highest peak, your levels of stress dropdown, better brain function will also help you get rid of any stress you might be having, and having overall better health can help you reduce weight. Overall, all the health benefits you get from intermittent fasting will help you get rid of your stress or at least lower it. This means, even if you are not facing pressure, intermittent fasting will help you have a better functioning brain and also help you get rid of any mental fog or anxiety you might be dealing with. What that in mind, always make sure you consult a physician if you are noticing much more stress than you can handle, as it can be something severe and not fixable by intermittent fasting.

Chapter 3: Different types of fasting protocol

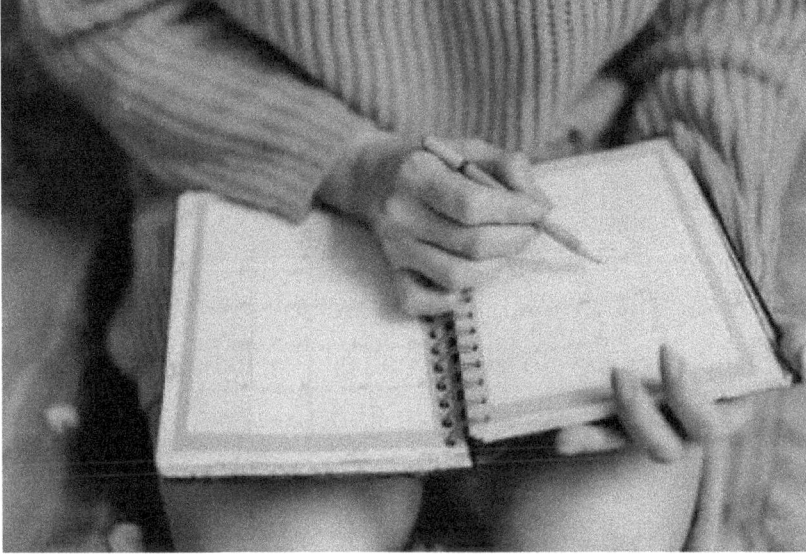

Glucose and fat are the two primary sources of energy for our bodies. Since glucose is more easily broken down than fat, our organization, by default, chooses glucose over fat when both are available. But, if glucose is not possible, the body can quickly turn to fat for its energy needs, and that too, without any harmful effect. At the fundamental level, intermittent fasting compels your body to burn off the excess fat into energy to meet its calorie requirements in the absence of food. What is body fat? It is nothing but excess energy from food that is stored away. If you don't consume, your body will 'eat' the stored fat for its energy needs. Insulin is one of the most critical hormones associated with food digestion.

The level of insulin in your bloodstream increases when you eat. Insulin facilitates the storage of food energy in two ways. First, simple sugars are converted into glycogen and stored in the liver. The liver may have resembled your refrigerator in which it is easy to store and access food, but there is limited space. Second, owing to limited storage space in the liver, glycogen gets converted into fat, which is then taken to other parts of the body and stored as fat deposits. The transfer and deposition of fat is a complex process. But there is no limit on the amount of fat that your body can store. Your body can be compared to a large freezer in which storing food is challenging to store and access. The food stored in that freezer will remain, and if not removed or taken care of, it can turn toxic, just like your fat deposits. The trick in any health-focused regimen, whether it is a diet or fast, is to work on and access the freezer. Therefore, there are two alternative sources of energy in our body.

One is in the form of glycogen (limited amount) in the liver, and the second one is in the way of fat deposits all over the body. The glycogen is easily accessible, whereas the fat is more difficult to access as it is spread all over the body. Now, when the body is in a fasting state, the level of insulin in the blood gets reduced. This reduction in insulin will signal the body to start burning stored energy to meet its energy requirements. The body does not receive food. The glucose level in the blood falls, which means the body will draw stored glycogen from the liver. When this stored glycogen supply is consumed, the body will turn to stored fat for its energy needs. Our organization, therefore, exists in only two states; the fed state where insulin levels are high and the fasting state where insulin levels are low.

In the fed state, our body is storing food energy, and in the fasting state, our body is burning this energy. It's always one state or the other. If we balance the fed and fasting rules, there will be no weight gain. Look at the typical modern-day scenario. We start eating from the minute we get up from sleep in the morning and continue to feed ourselves until we go back to sleep at night. This fed state is continuously storing food energy. There is very little fasting time given to the body to use up this stored energy. Your body will never get an opportunity to burn up the stored energy because you are regularly supplying it with food. There is no balance between the fed and the fasting state resulting in weight gain.

Intermittent fasting helps you regain the essential balance between the fed and the fasting states, thereby helping you lead a healthier life than before. During fasting rules, it is not only fats that are being broken. Realistically, our body uses a combination of lipids (from adipose tissues), ketones (from the fatty acids of the liver), and glucose made from glycogen (in liver and muscles) for its energy during the fasting state. All these forms of energy are needed because different tissues require different kinds of fuel: The muscles use the glucose from the glycogen stored in them for energy or fats from adipose fabrics.

The heart functions excellently with fats. Nerves and the brain prefer to work most efficiently with glucose though they can use ketones too. Red blood cells need only glucose and ketones, or they cannot use fatty acids. Therefore, the body requires to maintain sufficient blood-sugar levels for the RBCs to do their work and for the brain to function correctly. During fasting, this glucose has been converted and stored from the liver into sugar through a process called glycogenolysis. The liver is also capable of converting stored fat and amino acids into glucose. The method of metabolism in our body is quite complicated, and it is essential to remember that it needs all three macronutrients to function efficiently. Fasting empowers our metabolic system to leverage the power of stored fat for nearly all its energy purposes.

Types of Intermittent Fasting

There are various types of intermittent fasting, which is one of the reasons for its flexibility of use. Depending on your suitability, you can choose one or more methods. You could start with the easiest and most popular way, and slowly advance to more complicated options at your pace.

The 12-12 Method

This is the easiest and the most popular method of intermittent fasting and is perfect for beginners. You could already be in this schedule unwittingly. In this method, you have an eating window of 12 hours and a fasting window of 12 hours. So, if your dinner time is 8 pm and you have breakfast the next morning at 8 am, then you are already on this schedule, and you don't even know it. If you have been snacking after dinner, you should stop it immediately. For beginners, this method is excellent to get your body and mind strict about eating and feasting windows.

The 16:8

Method This is also achievable by most novices. However, it can be a massive challenge for people who don't like to miss dinner AND breakfast. The keyword here is 'AND.' For this method to be a success, you must be ready to skip one of these two meals. By skipping one of the two flours, you will get a 16-hour fasting window, which includes your 8-hour sleeping time. Your feeding window will be a balance of 8 hours a day. For people who have never fasted before, this method could be a high starting point. Finish your dinner by 8 pm and get to bed by 10 pm. When you wake up at 6 am the next morning, 10 hours of the fasting period is already done. Skip breakfast, and you can have your first meal of the day at noon. Just make sure you hydrate yourself well during the fasting window.

Also, you can drink tea or coffee, black and sugarless, which can help fight hunger pangs. Although initially, it might be tough, it does get more comfortable as you persist. During the feasting window, you can fit in 2 or 3 meals. This method is referred to as the Leangains protocol and was made accessible by Martin Berkhan, a famous fitness expert. The dinner-skipping way of following the Leangains process involves an eating window from 8 am – 4 pm (your last meal of the day) and a fasting window of 4 pm – 8 am the next day. If 4 pm for your previous lunch is very far away from your bedtime, you can shift your eating to 10 am (your first meal of the day) to 6 pm (your last meal of the day). Here is a small chart to help you understand how you can plan your 16:8 daily intermittent fasting schedules: If your first meal is at 7 AM, your last meal should be at 3 pm. If your first meal is at 8 AM, your last meal should be at 4 pm. If your first meal is at 11 AM, your last meal should be at 7 pm. If your first meal is at 2 PM, your last meal should be at 10 pm. The 18:6 Method This method will test your willpower a little more than the 16:8 process. It is more challenging to achieve than the previous way as you need to gather all your mental strength and fight off hunger pangs for 18 hours; 2 hours more than 16! Moreover, with an eating window of only 6 hours, you cannot get more than two meals, and perhaps, squeeze in one little snack in-between. The good thing about this method is once you have perfected it and your body and mind have come to accept it as part of your life, you don't have to try any more extreme intermittent fasting methods.

The 18:6 method

Will suffice for the rest of your life. You can extend each day's fasting regimen to cover more hours for fasting and lesser hours for eating. For example, you could have a fasting window for 20 hours and an eating window of 4 hours (20:4, tough yes, but doable over a long period). Or, you could have one meal a day in which you ensure you get all the nutrients your body needs. The last two methods are extreme and cannot be done daily. You can keep them for special days to test your mental strength and willpower capacity. Even the keenest fasting advocates might not be able to manage the 20:4 and one-meal-a-day consistently. Additionally, any extreme fasting method to be maintained for more than a couple of days should never be attempted without medical supervision.

The 5:2 Diet

This method of intermittent fasting entails following a healthy eating pattern (without any fasting schedule) on five days of the week and restricting calorie intake to 500-600 calories on two days. This diet is called the Fast Diet and was made famous by Michael Mosley, a British doctor, and journalist. Women are advised to consume 500 calories and men 600 calories on the two fasting days of the week. A great example of the 5:2 diet would be to restrict calorie intake on Mondays and Thursdays, and generally eating on all the other days. You can choose any two days that are suitable for you. However, the most effective way of doing this fast is to choose two consecutive fasting days when you will restrict your calorie intake to 500-600. Your metabolism will highly benefit from this method of fasting, especially if you can manage two consecutive fasting days instead of two separate days.

The 24-Hour Fast

While eating one meal a day regularly is not just difficult but also not highly advised, fasting one day a week for 24 hours is doable and a great intermittent fasting method too. Brad Pilon, another famous fitness expert, advocated and popularized this method of intermittent fasting. Dinner at 7 pm on Monday, followed by dinner at 7 pm on Tuesday, is an example of the 24-hour fasting method. You could also choose to do breakfast-to-breakfast or lunch-to-lunch. During the 24-hour fasting period, only tea, coffee, and other non-calorie liquids are allowed. The trick to making a success of this intermittent fasting method is to stick to generally eating on your first meal after the 24-hour fasting period. You must consume the same amount of food that you would have eaten had you not fasted. Again, staying in the fasting mode for 24 hours can be a considerable challenge for many. The first few hours might go off uneventfully, but later on, ravenous hunger can create a lot of temporary discomforts. You will have to give your best self-discipline ways to make this method a success. However, you don't need to start in such a rigorous way. Instead of starting at the 24-hour level, you can begin with a 14-16-hour level on one day of the first week, and slowly increase it to 24 hours after 3-4 weeks or at your pace. The Alternate-Day Fasting Method This method requires you to fast every other day and usually eat every other day. On the fasting days, your calorie intake should be restricted to 500-600. The alternate-day fasting method calls for going hungry to bed several days each week, which may not be an easy or pleasant thing to do and can be quite an extreme method.

The Warrior Diet

This method of intermittent fasting entails consuming: Fruits and raw vegetables in small quantities during the day. One big meal at dinner time. Primarily, the warrior diet consists of fasting all day and feasting at one feast. However, it is different from the rigorous 24-hour fasting diet because here, you do consume fruits and vegetables, which can be great to stave off hunger pangs effectively and in a healthy manner.

The nighttime meal is typically similar to the paleo diet consisting of wholesome and unprocessed foods that are as close to how nature provides them as possible. Despite the fruits and vegetables, the Warrior Diet can be quite a challenge. As beginners, it might not make sense to try it until you have understood how your body responds to more straightforward methods of intermittent fasting. Spontaneous Intermitting Fasting This method does not have any structure or planning for it. You choose to skip one or two meals if you are not feeling hungry or do not have the time to cook, or you feel like it or for any other reason.

Having to eat regularly to remain energized and active is nothing but a myth. The fear of entering 'starvation mode' looms so large that we end up eating far more than what we need. Our body is well-equipped to manage not just missing a couple of meals but times of great famine. So, if you do not feel hungry, don't hesitate to skip a couple of meals. Just be conscious of not overeating when you do sit down to your meal after a couple of skips. Also, stick to healthy foods during your mealtimes. The trick in intermittent fasting is to cut calorie intake by cutting down the number of meals. Skipping meals whenever you feel inclined is referred to as spontaneous intermitting fasting. The flip side of this method is a lack of plan and strategy that could lead you to become irreverent and undisciplined in your approach leading to ineffective results. However, if you are a naturally disciplined person and have ingrained the habit of intermittent fasting into your system, then the spontaneous method will work correctly.

The water fast

Well, the name says it all; this method has got to be one most laborious fasting methods that you can follow. Most of the ways can be used for an extended period, but I would suggest this method is only used only certain times a year. I would only use this method as a tool rather than a lifestyle, as doing this for too long can do some damage to your body. That being said, this method can be used to your advantage, but first, let's talk about how this method works.

This method is based on you eating like you usually would, and then fasting for one to three days with the only thing that you can have during your fasting period is water. The best way to start this fast is to plan it ahead of time, slowly lower the calories every day as you get closer to your pool fast as it will prepare your body, and it won't be such a shock. An example will be if you were consuming two thousand calories day, what I would recommend is to lower five hundred calories every day, so on the fourth day, you can start your fast without it being a shock. Now the best way to go about fasting is to fast for one to two days no longer than three days, some people have fasted for ten days using this method, but I would not recommend you go without food for that long, and I don't see the reason why you should be fasting for so long. Since there are not a lot of guidelines on how often should you fast using this method, the best way would be to use this method is to fast every four to eight weeks, and I wouldn't go past three days of actual fasting. I would recommend you fast on days that you are not doing anything physically like working out since it can affect your workout and your whole day after that. One thing I would recommend you don't do is to use this method more than twelve times in a year, as doing it often can affect your day to day life and energy levels based on experiences. Although this method can't be used as a lifestyle, there are some benefits to these methods, so let's talk about them.

This method is best known for cleaning out toxins in your body. Since you won't eat for one to three days and the only thing that you will be consuming is water, your body will automatically get rid of toxins in your body with the help of water. This has got be a selling point for me when it comes to using this method, don't get me wrong every fasting method helps with cleaning out your body, but if your body doesn't ingest anything for one to three days, then that gives your body plenty of time to "clean up." Another fantastic benefit of using this method is that it will clean out any harmful bacteria in your gut, which will help you digest your food better the next time you consume some. Since you will be getting rid of toxins in your body, you will also get the benefit of lowered risk of diseases, which is always a plus. Another thing this method can help you with is a fat loss since you won't be eating for so long your body will depend on fat for energy, but I would not use this method for fat loss as there are other methods that you can use for that goal. As you can see, this method has some benefits, now let us talk about some issues that you can have with this method.

The first issue with this method is that it can be super hard to go thru with. Fasting for one to three days with no food requires a lot of will power, and often, people won't go thru with this method since it's so hard. Another issue that this method could have is that it can affect your strength, if you are into strength training then be prepared to lose some strength following this plan to often, This issues can be kept in control if you fast on non-workout days and use this method every four to eight weeks. One of the major flaws with this method is that there is a chance that you can go hypoglycemic, so be careful as this can get super dangerous if you fast for an extended period. These are the main issues with using this method, most of the problems can be fixed if you be careful and don't use this method often meaning not exceeding more than three days of fasting and easing into the technique.

The Positives of Intermittent

Fasting If you plan your meals to fit into a smaller eating window, you are more likely to be a conscious eater than if you choose to leave the entire day open to eat whenever you like. With intermittent fasting, you tend to become a more mindful eater than before. Eating mindlessly is one of the biggest causes of binge-eating. Another thing about intermittent fasting is that while you have to keep a general control over calorie intake, you don't have to micromanage this aspect.

Therefore, given the freedom to eat what you want (in reasonable amounts) could drive you to consume healthier foods. Many times, excessive restrictions encourage us to do something we should not do. Intermittent fasting gives you a reasonable amount of freedom to eat your favorite foods during your eating window. The Negatives of Intermittent Fasting For some people, the fact that you can eat whatever you want can be counterproductive because they end up binge-eating at every meal during the eating window. This approach will end up defeating the core desire of intermittent fasting, and you could eat far more than needed resulting in weight gain and an unhealthy lifestyle.

The initial hiccups could drive some people to overreact to hunger pangs and cravings, resulting in cultivating worse eating habits than before. All the initial setbacks of intermittent fasting and how to cope with them are discussed in greater detail. Moreover, restricting the time of eating could also make some people think that it is another form of 'diet.' This dieting mindset can be detrimental to achieving your intermittent fasting goals. A necessary mindset of 'following a diet' will make you less likely to follow through the process than you look at it as an altered eating pattern. The most important thing you must remember about intermittent fasting is that it is not a crash diet that you can try for 3-5 days before an upcoming party to fit into a dress you've bought for yourself. It is a choice of a lifetime to change the way you eat for the rest of your life. Read on for more benefits, cautionary advice, and more about intermittent fasting.

Chapter 4: How to Pick the Right Plan Based on Your Lifestyle

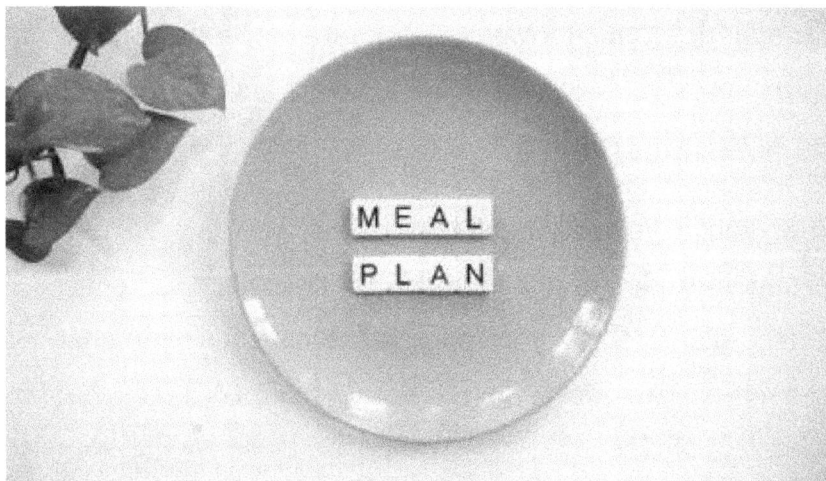

In this chapter, we will help you understand how to pick out the right plan when it comes to intermittent fasting protocol. One thing to realize would be that intimate fasting can be customized based on your needs. If you are someone looking to have eating schedules based on your lifestyle, then chances are intermittent fasting is the answer for you. As you know, by now, there are tons of ways for you to follow intermittent fasting. We talked about the different intermittent fasting protocols, and which one will benefit you in what way. One thing to remember is that you will still see many of the benefits we discussed in the previous chapters, regardless of the plan you follow. Which means that following intermittent fasting or certain protocol should not demotivate you when it comes to following a certain plan. With that being said, what we will do in this chapter is it go through different Lifestyles and how certain intermittent fasting protocols will work in a much better way when it comes to seeing success with intermittent fasting.

Now, you have to remember that we can only go through certain lifestyles and scenarios. Don't expect us to have a perfect scenario for you. You will have to decide that for yourself, and once you're done reading this chapter. However, all the scenarios should be close to the scenario you are living in. also, if we suggest a certain intermittent fasting protocol based on the scenarios, make sure that you still try on all the intermittent fasting protocols and realize which one works for you. The truth is, the best personal trainer is the best nutritionist you're going to have you. Once you start understanding your body, then you will be in a much better position of not only utilizing intermittent fasting at its full potential, but you also have a great idea off went to stop and when you should begin.

If that makes sense, then you should be steps ahead of your trainers and nutritionists, which you might hire. We are not saying that you should not have a personal trainer or nutritionist, what we are saying is that you will be in a much better position if you can understand how your body functions to create a customized plan for you. Now the first scenario we are going to be using would be very similar to someone who works in a nine-to-five job. If your someone who works from 9 to 5 and only gets one lunch break during the day and chances are 16/ 8, intermittent fasting would be ideal for you. To clarify, you can always start with a 12/12 intermittent fasting protocol, in the beginning, to get ready. However, once you get your feet wet with intermittent fasting, then you should go with the 16/8 method.

The reason why the 16/8 method works so well for people who work a 9to five job it is because it is straightforward to manage. The beauty of the 16/8 method when it comes to intermittent fasting is that you can set the hours to whatever time you want to eat, and you don't want to eat. For example, many people notice better brain functioning when they are not eating any food. This means you can skip breakfast and not eat throughout the whole workday allowing you to focus on the task at hand. Then once you're done working, you can have yourself a nice big breakfast. We know numerous amounts of people doing this, and not only did the notice they lost a lot of weight, but they also got a lot better at the work which they are performing. The beauty of intermittent fasting would be that it allows you to not only lose body fat but give you the mental clarity that you're looking for.

The reason why you get mental Clarity is that you will not be spiking up your insulin throughout the day. When you spike up your insulin, you will notice things such as lethargy and overall laziness. This is why the 16/8 method works so great when it comes to recovering any issues which you might be facing when it comes to mental fog or mental fatigue. That being said, start with the 12/12 method and slowly build-up to the 16/8 method to see better results. In this scenario, not only will your work performance go up, but you also lose a lot of weight and get the overall health benefit that you're looking for when it comes to intermittent fasting. This will work especially well for people who are above the age of 50.

The reason why it will work a lot better for people who are above the age of 50 is simply that they will go through a phase known as autophagy. As you know, autophagy has been shown to reduce many health complications, including the slowing down of aging. This makes it ideal for people looking to slow down aging. So if you work a nine-to-five job and you're looking to lose body fat while slowing down aging, then we highly recommend that you follow the 16/8 method throughout the workday. Meaning fastest route to the workday, and have yourself a nice breakfast after you're done working. I want you to perform a lot better at your workplace, and to see better results overall when it comes to intermittent fasting and losing body fat. Keep in mind, the scenario we just talked about is the first scenario that most people will be going through.

However, we have a ton of scenarios to talk about. now chances are there will be a lot of people who work in labor, looking to reap the benefits of intermittent fasting. Now, if you are working labor, chances are it will be a little bit more difficult for you to continue with intermittent passing. However, with the right scheduling in the right planning, you should have no problem concerning intermittent fasting. now let's say you work the labor 8 hours a day. What we would recommend is trying to have most of your calories throughout the 8-hour window. Once you are done with your work, make sure that you start your fast right away.

Now there are a lot of ways for you to get your calories throughout your eating window while you are working. You can have things such as protein shake, and You are quickly you going to have a pre-prepared meal, which will help you to consume all the calories you need throughout the whole day. The reason why we recommend you eat throughout the day while you're working is that a labor job could be tedious. We want to make sure that you don't paint or affect your work in any way possible. This is why we recommend you follow the 16 by eight method and include your eating window while you are working. Many people who work in labor tend to follow this protocol, the reason why it works so well. That's because they won't get all the calories they need when they need it. you need to have a good steady flow of food intake while you are physically working.

Your body can only break down fat so quickly, which is why a good amount of carbohydrates and nutrients is important when you're performing anything physical. That being said, you can always resort to the 5/2 method when you are intermittent fasting. If you don't like the 16/8 method, then you can always follow the 5/2 method. This method works great as you only have to "fast" for two days out of the week, meaning you can normally eat when you are working. As you get older, especially in the labor workforce, you will be required to be well-fed when you're working. The last thing we want is for you to have injuries at your workplace. That being said, you can either follow the 16/8 method, or you can go right ahead and follow the 5/2 method fasting on your non-working days.

This will allow you to see the results that you're looking for when it comes to anti-aging, regardless of the fasting protocol you follow. However, if we're honest, the 16/8 method works a lot better when it comes to seeing results in regards to intermittent fasting and anti-aging. Now let's pick out another scenario, what's talked about someone who works the night shift. If you're someone who works the night shift, the chances are that you will be in a much better scenario than a lot of people. The reason why you will be in a much better position than a lot of people is that nightshift tends to be slow for most cases. Now, if you're a nurse, then chances are you will have no time to eat any food.

So the best thing for you to do would be not to have any food during your shift, and once you're done your shift, you can have more food allowing you to be a lot better at fasting. The great thing about being a nurse or working a night shift would be that you will have a much better position of not only continued with intermittent fasting but the desire to not eat. Numerous times we have heard nurses talk about not having the time to eat, or simply not in the mood for eating anything. Having this mentality will help you tremendously to continue with intermittent fasting, which is why it is so important to understand which intermittent fasting protocol works for your needs. Batting said if your nurse is working night shifts, the best-case scenario for you would be too fast brought your whole shift and have your eating window once you're done your work. For instance, let's say you work 10 hours a day, then fast for 10 hours a day and eat for the remainder of the time. This gets a little bit tricky for a nurse, as the hours can be scattered or sometimes not be ideal case scenario for you too fast. However, the best way to go about fasting if your nurse who is who works a shift at a very demanding job, we recommend you fast during the time you are working. This will allow you to be in a perfect position when it comes to fasting and to see the best results overall with intermittent fasting. In essence, you will be trying out all the types of intermittent fasting when you are working the night shift or working as a nurse, for example. Depending on your shift, you will be fasting either 10 hours or even up to 24 hours, depending on how you feel. That being said, this will give you the best possible scenario for you to continue with intermittent fasting and to make it a habit. Many people don't realize it, but making intermittent fasting a part of your life is much more important than someone looking to follow a specific plan. Now we have given you enough scenarios to figure out which plan would work best for you based on your lifestyle. Now we will move on and talk about all the methods and which deliver the specific goal that you're looking for. Keep in mind that all these plans will work tremendously well if you're looking to slow down aging and to lose body fat overall feeling better about yourself. However, we will break down all the plans so that you have a better idea of which one to pick and finalize.

16/8: As you know, the 16/8 method is one of the most popular ways when it comes to intermittent fasting. The 16/8 way will not only help you to lose body fat, but it will also help you with the anti-aging process and to better your overall function. Many people follow the 16/8 method as it is the most convenient method to follow and comfortably flexible. Depending on your lifestyle, this method could work very well when it comes to giving you the results that you're looking for. The beauty of this method is that you can build muscle, lose fat, and do anything you want while making this a life choice. When I say a life choice, it means that you can follow this plan for the rest of your life and not feel taxed out. If it is feasible for you, then we highly recommend that you follow the 16/8 method, one of the most studied ways of intermittent fasting.

12/12: Now, this method is for someone who's looking to set up intermittent fasting without going too hard if you don't know how intermittent fasting works or you don't know if it is going to be the right path for you then you should start with the 12/12 method. This method will allow you to get your feet wet when it comes to intermittent fasting so that you can continue with intermittent fasting if you enjoy it or make it a little bit more challenging by upping the fasting times. That being said, but 12/12 method is merely something to get your feet wet with and not something you should do for the rest of your life. The secure trolls method is a great plan to start. However, you will not see the anti-aging effects or the weight loss effects that you're looking for following this method. In the beginning, you will, however, as you go along, you will not see the results that you are looking for when it comes to losing body fat are slowing down the aging process. This is where the 16/8 method will shine, as it will give you sufficient time to fast while seeing the benefits that you are hoping to get out of intermittent fasting.

The water fast: Now the water fast is for someone who is looking to not only detoxify their body, but they're changing the way their body functions. This plan is only to be followed a handful of times to detoxify their gut, so they digest a lot better. If you might know, the stomach is known as the second brain. The reason why it is known as a second brain is that your body heavily depends on your gut and how it digests, as you know, eating food as necessary for a livelihood, which is why we must take care of the organs, especially our gut. Make sure you use this method to clean out your organs and to see better results from it. This will allow you to be in a better position when it comes to digesting food and keeping your organs beautiful and safe.

5:2 Diet: This fasting protocol is ideal for people who are looking to lose weight quickly, now if you're someone who wants to lose weight rapidly and has a motivation and willpower to get it done then the 5/2 works the best. A disciple makes you lose a lot of body fat and a short period, allowing you to live a lot better life overall. Now keep in mind that following the 5/2 diet will not help you with any anti-aging process in the long-term. But I will help you detoxify your body and to make you lose a ton of weight, especially in the beginning. Don't follow this protocol for the rest of your life as it is not sustainable. However, once you get the hang of this plan, you will be in a much better position to lose fat and to get your goal weight a lot quicker than you would. Once you've lost a way to find the 5/2 diet, we recommend that you started following the 16/8 diet quickly. The 16/8 diet is where you want to be when it comes to see long-lasting results. Regardless of the 5/2 diet will work for you if you do a labor job, because of the structure.

This chapter should give you a clear idea of how intermittent fasting works and which protocol you should be following when it comes to bettering your results based on your lifestyle. Now some people might find this chapter very basic or vague. Keep in mind that we want you to use your brain when it comes to picking out the right plan. If you remember in the beginning, we told you that the best nutritionist or the trainer for you would be yourself, which is why we need you to understand this chapter and pick up the plan which works for your lifestyle and your goals. As always, make sure that you know your body before you start following any of these plans. We recommend a start off with a 12/12 method as you will see significant benefits from it in the beginning. However, once you get your feet wet with intermittent fasting, then we recommend that you start following other plans that will help you achieve that goal as well.

Chapter 5: How Does Intermittent Fasting Slow Down Aging

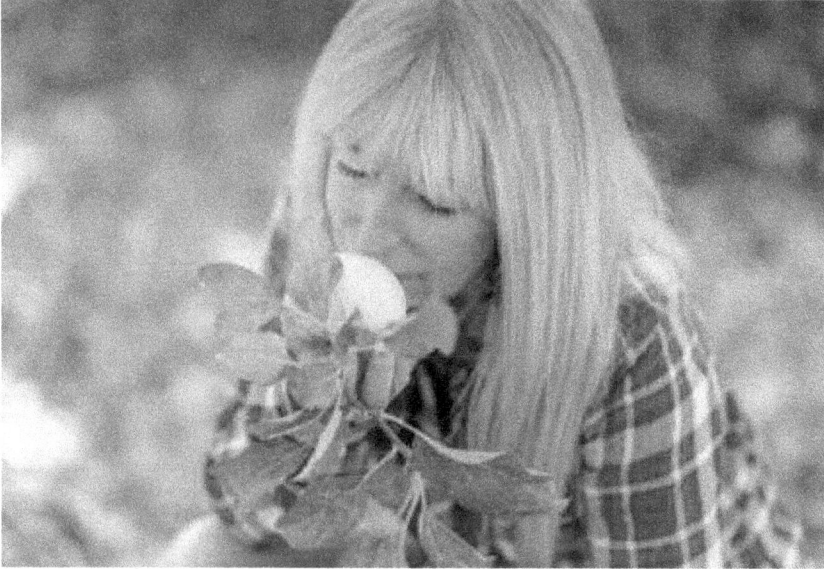

When we were kids, it sometimes felt like we couldn't wait to grow up, so we didn't have to listen to our parents. Even when we graduated high school, we might have wished we could be even older so we could drink alcohol, have a better job, and just more freedom in general. Once you hit a certain age, you start to realize that as you get older time goes by faster each year as well. Not only this, but it's harder to keep up with your health. You might have been able to eat nothing but potato chips and ice cream in a day and felt fine, but that same kind of meal now could sound like a night of indigestion. We can never reverse aging, and until we have a time machine, there's no going back. You will always be as old as you've ever been, and as young as you will ever be, the rest of your life, each moment that you live. This kind of thinking can be terrifying, but it's also important to remember as we choose the right type of diets for our health. The better choices you make, the longer your life can be. There will always be certain unavoidable things and accidents which can change our plans, however, that doesn't mean we shouldn't be trying to live as long as possible, as healthy as we can be. *Reducing the Stress Hormone Levels: An increase in insulin levels can also be directly affected by our stress levels. When we feel stressed out, our bodies release cortisol. This hormone is necessary to provide energy to our muscular system. When you're stressed, your body will go into a flight/fight mode, which helps protect you against this threat felt. This is why you might notice your shoulders are sore when you're stressed, or that you keep your jaw and fists clenched, resulting in some muscle fatigue. This release of cortisol can also mean a higher level of glucose throughout your bloodstream. If you are stressed out all the time, then this means you are continually releasing that cortisol, steadily increasing your blood sugar. Stress that results in no physical activity isn't good either, because then you're just holding onto that energy. If we want to reduce our insulin levels and keep our body regulated, then stress needs to be managed as well* (Kresser, 2019).

Lowering the Insulin Levels As you get older, it's harder to keep up with your health. Even those who actively try to eat healthily and the workout will find that they struggle a lot more in their older years than they did when they were young and healthy teens. Those at any age who eat unhealthily are at risk of forming insulin resistance and certain types of diabetes. Diabetes is much more common in older individuals, meaning if we want to keep our health long throughout our lives, we need to focus on regulating insulin right now. We already discussed how fasting could control your insulin and keep you from becoming insulin resistant, so no need to explain that again here.

What's important to remember, however, is that you should always consider an increase in your insulin sensitivity as you get older. It's not easy to accept, but our health will only get more challenging to manage, so we need to focus on doing that now so we can live a long and happy life. Keeping Your Liver Healthy One thing we haven't talked about, yet very much is your liver, and how this can affect your health. You might instantly think about alcohol when it comes to your liver, knowing that too much alcohol can have adverse effects on this. However, your liver is responsible for a lot more than just processing the alcohol you drink. A detox of your liver can help in your process of losing weight. However, after you've gone through rehab, then you need to keep up with a healthy lifestyle, or else your liver will be subjected to the same things. The thing about your liver is that this is the part of your body that helps detoxify! It is your body's filtration system, helping to remove toxins throughout your body. While it is mighty and even capable of regenerating itself, you still need to treat it right, giving it as few toxins to get rid of as possible. The first toxin that you will run into is additives to any processed foods. This is going to include things like food dyes and artificial flavors that aren't typically meant for regular consumption.

Alternatively, consider other chemicals, pesticides, and hormones that are added to processed foods, which could directly affect the efficiency of your liver. Intermittent fasting is an excellent choice for your liver because it is a process to detox your body. Think of it like giving your liver a little break from its job. As you process fatty stored cells during a fast, these are simple things already broken down once in your body, meaning that when your liver does have to do work, it will be easier than what it might have been subjected to in the past. As we get older, we'll start to get more sensitive to other kinds of illnesses, meaning our filtration system will need to improve. There's no better time to start taking care of your liver than now (Browning, 2012). How to Use Fasting for Longevity Fasting promotes a healthier lifestyle and encourages better habits. Since it is a natural way to lose weight, it will last you longer. You could try out a complicated diet involving meal replacements and supplements, but at the end of the day, this might result in you gaining weight faster than you lost it. The fluctuation of weight gain and loss isn't always right on our bodies. To live a long and healthy life, you have to make healthy choices. Train your body to burn fat and detoxify continually, and you will be doing your very best to try and achieve longevity through the use of fasting.

Autophagy is when cells can clean themselves. It involves the process of a cell removing the toxins and other unwanted substances that might have penetrated their makeup. This would need to be done when a virus, harmful bacteria, or other poison has made its way into the body, regardless of the type of intruder versus cell attacked (Murrell, 2018). Whenever a foreign particle might be present, then your cells will be able to fight that or remove it using autophagy. Autophagy occurs throughout the day without us having any idea what's happening. Your body is smart, so just because you're adding things to it that are damaging doesn't mean that it's always going to feel those effects.

Our bodies aren't perfect, however, so they will still need some help through other processes that can kickstart or encourage autophagy. *Cleaning of Waste Cells and Pathogens: The stronger the cell, the better it will be able to clean waste and get rid of various pathogens in the body. Fasting is a great way to encourage autophagy and cause your cells to not only rid themselves of toxins but to repair new, stronger ones as well* (Murrell, 2018). You might notice some detoxes are doing things aimed at specific detoxification, such as a liver detox, a heart detox, or even a brain detox. This isn't necessary, as encouraging autophagy throughout your body will help work to clean it starting from the inside and eventually spreading throughout your body. *Stop Progression of Diseases: Autophagy could even help encourage the reduction of cancer cells, or at least help to prevent them from growing in the first place* (Bhutia, 2013). We have numerous mitochondria throughout our bodies that get older with time. Once they get to a certain age, they will start to release free radicals in our collection. These could end up causing mutations, sometimes mortal. To produce new mitochondria and rid ourselves of the old, then we will need to focus on encouraging autophagy within our bodies. Caloric restriction is the best way to reduce this at first. This isn't a cure-all, but caloric restriction has been helped to slow down the production and growth of various tumors (Murrell,

2018). This can be very specific, so you mustn't assume fasting is going to cure cancer. It might help prevent and reduce, but it's not necessarily a cure-all. To avoid it in the first place, encourage autophagy within your cells.

How Autophagy Impacts You

Autophagy will have many other benefits to your health that are important to understand. It helps with reducing the amount of stored fat, which is a benefit in itself while also helping to prevent other health conditions associated with being overweight. It can help repair damaged cells, which is essential to keep up productivity from where those cells are damaged. For example, if some cells in your stomach are damaged from a life of unhealthy eating, autophagy could help to repair those. All of this will also help reduce inflammation, which can have other serious health risks as well. When you experience redness, it can slow down specific processes and cause your organs to not work as well, depending on where the inflammation is present.

When you get a cut, it turns red and swells – this is inflammation. When we damage our bodies inside, they will become inflamed; we won't see it. This could have adverse health effects, such as sore and tight joints, slow-working systems (such as a digestive system that isn't working correctly/causes pain to use), and could even cause depression through an inflamed brain (Raison, 2011). If you don't have autophagy within your body's function, it puts you at risk for some cardiovascular, rheumatological, atherosclerosis, and pulmonary diseases. You might also be at a higher risk of cancer, holding onto more fat, muscle loss, and even sensitivity to the sun. Protein Cycling One way to induce autophagy is to use protein cycling. This is the process of having some higher amounts of protein during some phases and lowers at others. When fasting, it will be best to reduce your protein intake on the days that you are restricting your food. On your days of eating and no fasting, then you can go back to a reasonable amount of protein. Fasting days stick to 25 grams or less.

Other days, you can go back to normal, which is 46-56 grams depending on your sex/body weight. The point of keeping yourself from overeating protein will be to force your body to look elsewhere for its energy source. When Autophagy and Protein Cycling Matter Especially for Women These processes are essential to include even in those that don't want to lose weight because autophagy will reduce over time and become less efficient as we get older. This is especially important for women because we are at risk for certain estrogen-related diseases and cancers, and we usually have a higher fat content than the average healthy man. We want autophagy to work for us, and to reduce our body's toxins continually, so ensure that you are regulating your autophagy effectiveness through intermittent fasting. We already know by now that fasting will make your cells turn on themselves, fat being burned along the process.

Autophagy is your body's natural way of doing this, so it's clear to see that incorporating fasting will help to kickstart that natural process that already exists. Autophagy occurs within the first 24 hours of fasting, on average. This means that you aren't fasting for 24-hours, but you've restricted your caloric intake.

How to Induce Autophagy Through Intermittent Fasting

You might see supplements, teas, or other products that claim they induce autophagy. Still, the only obvious way that's proven to be safe and effective is to do it naturally through fasting. As you fast, you are lowering your insulin levels. Therefore, you have a higher chance of starting autophagy within your body. What's most important to induce autophagy is focusing on reducing your glycogen levels, which only shows after around 14 hours of fasting. For longer health, you will want to include extended periods of fasting for weeks, but preferably, months, at a time.

Chapter 6: How Should Women Fast Over 50?

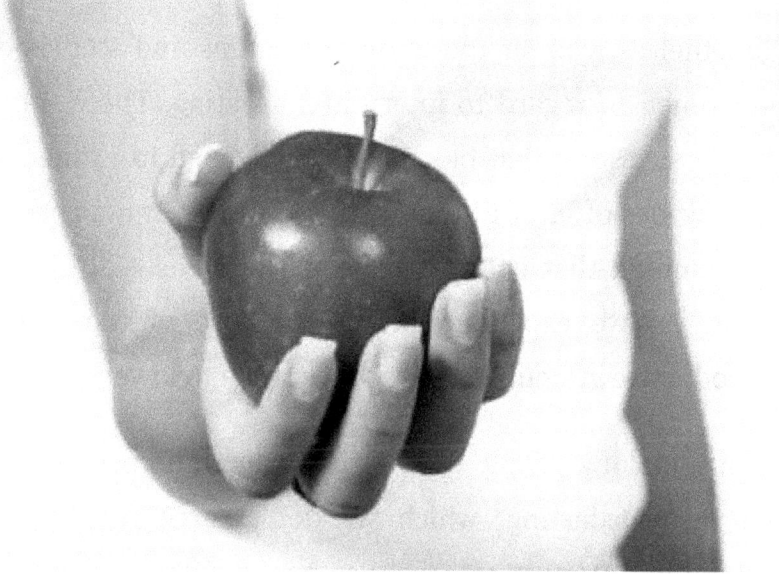

As we mentioned to you previously, intermittent fasting does not yield drastically different results in both men and women. However, there are many differences in regard to how women should follow intermittent fasting. The great news is that women can take part in all the fast's listed in this book, regardless we need to talk about intermittent fasting for women.

Some claims are suggesting that intermittent fasting needs to be modified, which is true to a certain degree if women use the easier going fasting protocols, which are available to review in the previous chapters. Then they should have no problem with intermittent fasting, and the problems start to occur when 48 hours+ fasts begin to take place.

Nonetheless, you should know the claims and studies done on women in regard to intermittent fasting. There was one study suggesting that blood sugar worsened in women after three weeks of intermittent fasting. Moreover, many sources are claiming that changes in women's menstrual cycle will occur. As we explained before, because of the woman's reproductive system, they are susceptible to lower calories.

Hence, making people believe that women do not indulge in intermittent fasting, which we don't agree with. If done tastefully, intermittent fasting has resulted in excellent health and weight loss benefits for women. So in this chapter, we will go thru exactly how occasional fasting affects women in all aspects, such as hormones, hunger craving, and many more things are on the agenda. With that in mind, let's get into the nitty-gritty.

The key to intermittent fasting for women in autophagy

You might have heard of autophagy in this book so far, now let me explain to you what autophagy truly means. Autophagy is a biological process that comes to the Greek word "auto," meaning "self" and "phagy," meaning "eat." It is a process where our body cleans out the bad cells and replace them with newer healthy ones, which is excellent for anyone looking to live a healthier life.

But sometimes, our body cannot get this process going for hosts of reasons. Mainly because we eat the food we can't digest properly, which makes our body work extra hard to cope up with the food instead of getting rid of "bad cells." As we get older, the process becomes less efficient. One of the proven ways to fix this issue, especially for women, is by fasting for 12 or more hours and allowing your body to focus more on getting rid of the "bad cells" by replacing them with newer and stronger ones.

This method works exceptionally well, especially on women, to rejuvenate their cells and to see the health benefits. The great news about autophagy is that you don't need to fast for an indefinite amount of time to notice the results, 12 to 16 hours of fast will do. This means women don't need to put yourself at risk by fasting for a prolonged period; this makes intermittent fasting a tool for women looking to stay young for more extended periods.

Remember that autophagy should not be just for anti-aging purposes, as it can help you with hosts of things. Consider autophagy as a detox for your whole body, and believe it or not; most people need it. Forget cleansing diets, and if you truly want to detox your body, then you need to fast for at least 12 hours a day.

For women, 12-16 hours should not result in adverse effects. You will also reduce the risk of cancer because you will have newer and stronger cells at your disposal; another great benefit would be the fact that your metabolism will go up helping you with weight loss.

All in all, promoting the process of autophagy a great way to encourage better health, especially for women. Having healthier cells in a women's body will help you by having a better reproductive system, and you will have a higher chance of conceiving. Even though these claims haven't been backed up, it is still good to know that some excellent benefits come with intermittent fasting for women.

Finally, you will notice benefits such as better skin, better digestion of more energy throughout the day. To see the best results, fast for 12 to 16 hours a day, three times a week.

Make sure you space out your days, instead of doing all the fasts back to back. If you want to fast through the week as many do, then make sure not to prolong it for more than 6-8 weeks.

Fasting and female hormones

Intermittent fasting has shown to affect females' hormones, and there are some things women need to consider before they start fasting. Some studies are showing how intermittent fasting can negatively impact the female's reproductive system, and the reason why these shifts occur is that women are sensitive to lower calorie intake. When the calories are low for women, a small part of the brain known as the hypothalamus is affected.

Hypothalamus can disrupt the production of gonadotropin-releasing hormone (GnRH), which is responsible for releasing the two reproductive hormones, luteinizing hormone (LH) and follicle-stimulating hormone (FSH). Once these hormones have been affected negatively from an extended period by restricting calories, you will be running a risk of irregular periods, infertility, poor bone health, and other health risks. Even though autophagy has shown to do the opposite, it puts women in a complicated situation when it comes to fasting. For that reason, we don't recommend women fast for more than 24 hours as it can affect women's hormones in a very drastic manner.

Instead, women should use a modified approach that we talked about in this book. To make sure women don't notice any hormone imbalance, fast alternate days instead of back to back, keeping you in a safe place. If you want to fast aggressively for weight loss, then our recommendation is not to prolong it for more than 4-6 weeks. But then again, make sure you consult a professional before you may start fasting as everybody is different. On the plus side, there are many benefits women will notice if they begin fasting the right way. As we know, heart disease is killing people every day, in one study done on obese women showed that intermittent fasting lowered LDL cholesterol or which is the leading cause of heart problems in North America.

Also, intermittent fasting has shown to make you more insulin sensitive. In one study of 100 obese women showed that six months of intermittent fasting reduced insulin levels by 29% and insulin resistance by 19 %, although blood sugar remained the same. Having higher sensitivity to insulin has shown to lower the risk of type 2 diabetes. Still, intermittent fasting may not be beneficial for women as it is for men in regards to blood sugar. In mice, it has been shown to increase longevity by 33%, although long term studies on humans are yet to be determined.

Finally, intermittent fasting can reduce inflammation levels. Even though more studies need to be executed for women and intermittent fasting, it is pretty clear that there are hosts of benefits if done right. As long as you are taking intermittent fasting the right way, and you are not abusing it, your hormones should be in check. Remember, if you are pregnant, this might affect you very differently. Moreover, we do not recommend women fast when they are pregnant or trying to conceive, but as long as you know the repercussions of fasting too long.

Why intermittent fasting affects women's hormones more than men's?

If you have been doing research online, then you might have read claims such as "intermittent fasting is not for women" or "if women intermittent fast, their hormones will be out of whack." This isn't the case, as we will discuss how intermittent fasting truly affects women's hormone as when compared to men.

To briefly talk about men, they were created to "hunt and gather" so to speak. Unlike women, they do not have to carry a baby, which is one of the reasons why intermittent fasting does not affect men as drastically as women. Women are more susceptive to hormones that are related to hunger, and the reason behind is women's reproductive system, as previously mentioned.

The good news is, it will not affect your thyroid as some "experts" will claim, women recognize hunger at a higher degree than men. We recently talked about the Hypothalamus gonadotropin-releasing hormone (GnRH), luteinizing hormone (LH), and follicle-stimulating hormone (FSH), which is responsible for making testosterone and sperm in men and triggering estrogen and ovulation in women.

Women tend to trigger these hormones differently when compared to men, and the main problem occurs because of kisspeptin. For readers that don't know what kisspeptin is, it is a protein-like molecule that neurons use to communicate with each other. Women tend to produce more kisspeptin when compared to men, which is a precursor to (GnRH).

As you know (GnRH) is going to dictate how women produce estrogen and how men are going to produce testosterone; another thing is that kisspeptin is very sensitive to the hunger hormone. If you remember, we mentioned that women are more vulnerable to the hunger hormone when compared to men? The reason behind this is kisspeptin, which causes women to produce less kisspeptin and leads to lower progesterone. In one study done on rats showed that when female rats fast for one day, which is more like a week for women, it caused them to lose 19% of their body weight, but their ovaries shrunk significantly.

Also, they noticed that female rats luteinizing hormone plummeted, and their estrogen levels went through the roof. To briefly touch upon thyroid, t3 levels were deceased. But, t3 levels are always decreasing between meals. The t4, which is responsible for producing thyroid, remained the same, which means the thyroid isn't being affected drastically. It is always suggested that you get regular blood work done to ensure your thyroid is fine, but one of them to tell if it isn't is by seeing how cold you get.

If you feel cold all the time, then the chances are your thyroid is lower. If you notice that you are getting starving throughout the day, and it becomes tough to fast, then break the fast and try it again later. As a woman, you need to listen to your more than men, as women tend to be more sensitive to hormones when intermittent fasting.

Eating enough calories

Since you now know the science behind intermittent fasting and how it can affect women's hormones, let us talk about eating enough calories, especially for women. Believe it or not, this is an important topic to discuss. Especially for women who are much more sensitive to hunger hormones or hormones in general when compared to men. Even though you might be fasting for weight loss, it is critical that you enough calories support your bodily function as a woman. Ideally speaking, women who are trying to lose weight should not eat bellow 200 calories of their maintenance, calculating your maintenance calories the formula is (bodyweight x 12).

Meaning, if your maintenance calories are 2,000 and you are looking to lose weight, then you should not cut it down less than 1,800. If you are someone looking to lose weight with intermittent fasting, we recommend having a macronutrient break down of 20% carbs 50% protein and 30% fats; this shows the percentage of calories coming from specific macronutrients.

We are keeping the carbs low to prevent insulin spikes in check if you are looking to lose weight, we want to keep the insulin as flatlined as possible. However, if you are someone looking to maintain weight and reap the health benefits of intermittent fasting, then we recommend having a macronutrient breakdown of 30% carbs 40% protein 30% fats since we have covered the calorie intake, lets briefly talk about the types of food you should be eating. What you eat to break your fast is just as essential as the number of calories you should be consuming. One thing you need to understand is not to go overboard on the fasting.

As you know, carbs tend to spike your insulin, and when you're fasting, your insulin levels are low, meaning whatever you eat, your body will be sensitive to it. Having spikes of insulin slows down fat loss. Therefore, lower insulin equals more fat burning. If you break your fast with higher amounts of carbs, you will be shutting down the fat burning process. Instead, what we recommend is eating two meals when you break into your eating window. The first one should be lower in carbs and higher in fats and protein; this will ensure you don't turn off your fat burning and get the most out of your fast. The second meal could be higher carbs, and this will help you get ready for the next day if you are fasting.

Another to remember is that your gut will be susceptible to high acidic foods such and drinks, so make sure you stick to foods that are less acidic when you break your fast. Greek yogurt, chicken with some veggies, or even soup works great to break your fast. Now whether your goal is to lose weight or live a healthier life, it is essential that you follow the right calorie intake and macronutrient intake. These tips will go a long way with both the criteria listed.

How to avoid feeling underfed

Since you now know how much to eat, let's talk about how to prevent feeling underfed. Believe it or not, both men and women notice this problem, which causes them to overeat. We need to make sure you don't feed underfed to avoid things like breaking a fast too soon or overeating. There is a couple of technique we can provide you with that shall help you with the feeling of underfed.

The first technique we recommend would be eating wholesome, healthy foods that have a lot of fiber in them. Even though you are free to eat whatever you want, it is still not recommended that you eat unhealthily. When you break your fast, the food you should be eating is high fiber, lower carbs, and moderate protein. What the fiber will do is help you feel fuller throughout the day, making you feel less underfed.

An example of this would be to eat more green leafy vegetables, as they will make you feel fuller for a long time. Since we are on the topic of plants, let us talk about vitamins, you need to have micronutrients dense meals when you are fasting. If you are feeling underfed when fasting, the chances are that you are not consuming enough vitamins and minerals, making you feel underfed.

Make sure you are getting your daily mineral intake during your eating window to avoid such adverse effects; you could take a vitamin supplement during your fasting window to obtain your minerals. But don't use the supplement to take care of your vitamin needs, make sure you are eating healthy foods instead of junk food to feel thoroughly fed. Also, drinking water for the whole day is essential. If you are not drinking enough water, then you have a much higher chance of feeling underfed.

Not only will the water help you feel fuller, but it will also help you to get rid of toxins in your body. Water is a must for a better fasting experience; another thing which can curb your hunger is coffee. If you drink black coffee during your fast, it will help you control any hunger cravings you might be having, which will make you feel less underfed.

One recommendation would be drinking your coffee during the earlier times of the day, instead of later. As drinking coffee then makes you crash pretty hard, which will make you crave more, so make sure you stay away from coffee later during the day. Perhaps consume your coffee earlier in the morning or before your workout works the best, but the main take away would be not to consume junk. Even though fasting allows you to eat whatever you want, it doesn't mean you should, as it can lead you feeling underfed and hungry in the long run. Make sure you are following all these steps to ensure not handling underfed, and as you know, women tend to experience more hunger.

How often should women follow intermittent fasting

When it comes to fasting, women are more sensitive than men. Hence, making the timings and the duration of fasting a bit more restricted than men. Experts suggest that women should have a more relaxed approach than men. This may include shorter fasting days, lesser fasting days, and sometimes eating some food during the fast. We always recommend women to not fast longer than 24 hours, that's why all the fasting protocols listed in this book have a fasting window of no more than 24 hours.

Also, whichever fasting protocol you decide to choose, make sure it is sustainable to you. As it can lead to fewer results overall and disappointment, these being the surface level issues. If women fast for longer than 24 hours, it can lead to hormones going out of whack, and you what could happen then. Another thing to make sure of would be to fast consecutive days in the beginning, and it is recommended that women fast three times a week on consecutive days to ensure they can handle it.

Follow this protocol for the first three weeks, and eventually, if your physician gives you the go, then start lasting longer. With that being said, some women should not follow intermittent fasting. If you are pregnant, trying to conceive, nursing, or under chronic stress, then fasting should not be done. This now brings me to the period women should fast for. Ideally, women should follow a fasting protocol for no longer than eight weeks.

It is ideal for women to take a break from internment fasting after fasting for eight weeks, women should take a whole week off from fasting ideally two weeks off. If you start to notice symptoms such as irregular periods, metabolic stress, anxiety, depression, and insomnia, then stop fasting right away and speak with your doctor. These could be a sign of fasting for too long, so make sure you are looking out for these symptoms every time. There are some fasts you should not do for a prolonged period, such as the 5:2 method and the alternate-day fasting.

For these two fasting protocols, make sure you are not exceeding the six-week mark of following it. Finally, women need to stay on alert when they are fasting, know your body, and make sure you feel right and healthy when you are fasting. Some hunger cravings are fine, but if you start to notice insanity high food cravings which you can't control no matter what, then it is safer to eat some food rather than put your hormones and body in danger.

Fasting can be very fragile in terms of improving health or deteriorating it, especially in women. Which means you need to make sure you ease into fasting and to take regular breaks from it. The timelines we recommend in this chapter works for most women, but consult with a professional before you start or stop a fasting protocol! Good luck.

Symptoms you should look out for

There are many signs to look for when intermittent fasting since you know most of the things related to intermittent fasting by now, let's talk about the significant symptoms to look for. The first one being hunger, many followers of intermittent fasting will notice insane amounts of desire when following intermittent fasting. Which is a given, since you will be going from eating four to six meals throughout the day to none.

The first couple of days will require a ton of willpower to get thru, but eventually, it will subside and get better in a week. Give it some time for your body to get used to intermittent fasting, and be aware of the fact that it will be a shock in the beginning. Besides hunger, cravings for food are very evident when following intermittent fasting. Chances of you breaking your fast will be very high, especially when you are just getting started with it. You will crave foods like a candy bar, fruits, soda's anything which will give you a ton of sugar quickly. You will have to fight these cravings as they will kick in, so make sure you don't indulge in them. Headaches are another thing which beginners might notice.

When you start your intermittent fasting, you will see symptoms such as headaches, don't get worried as they will subside in a week in most cases. Make sure you are drinking plenty of water during your fasting window and after, as this will make it easy for your body to cope with the headaches.

One of the main symptoms you should be looking out for would be feeling cold. You will be contacting cold for the first week, but if it continues past the three-week mark, then consider modifying your fasting protocol. Intermittent fasting has shown to increase blood flow to your fat stores for your body to use it for energy, but if you start feeling cold shivering past the three-week mark, then it is a symptom you should be looking out.

Since you will be drinking a lot of water, this will make you feel even colder throughout the day, so unless you feel cold, don't take it seriously. Speaking of drinking water, you will also notice you going to the bathroom a lot. It is because of your water consumption, and there isn't a way around it since we don't recommend you drink less water. These are the main symptoms you will notice when you first start intermittent fasting, and they usually last three weeks.

If you experience these symptoms at the same magnitude as you were the first week, then please modify your fasting protocol as it might not be suitable for your body. If you healthily want to follow intermittent fasting, then it is best to look out for these symptoms and to listen to your body. If you're going to avoid these symptoms, then ease into intermittent fasting and making sure it isn't a shock for your body from the get-go.

Tips for intermittent fasting for women

Let's talk about some quick tips women need to consider before they start intermittent fasting, as there are some great ones to find before you start. The first tip would be to drink a ton of water when fasting, pretty easy to follow and understand. You need to drink water to curb your cravings, as you know, women tend to crave foods more than men do only because of the hormone response.

Drinking water will also help you control the headache symptoms you might get; overall, drinking water is a must. Drinking tea and coffee will help you manage your hunger throughout the day; it will also give you more energy in the beginning stages of fasting.

Just make sure you drink black coffee or black/green tea, don't add any sugar or milk as it will break your fast if you do that. If you find yourself around people who aren't supportive of your fasting endeavors, then make sure you stay away from them or at least avoid talking about fasting. The last thing you want is unsupportive people when you are following intermittent fasting, so make sure you stay away from them and stay positive. Finally, give yourself at least a month when you start intermittent fasting.

Many people don't realize that it will take some time to start seeing changes in their body; four weeks is a good time for your body to begin adapting to intermittent fasting. Meaning, you need to keep up the fast for at least a month for you to make a judgment whether fasting is for you or not, and most of the time, it works out in your favor. In the first four weeks of fasting, you will notice hunger waves avoid them by drinking coffee or tea. The main tip when intermittent fasting would be to not binge eat when you break your fast, you will have the craving to binge eat.

Avoid it. Follow our macros and eating patterns, which we have listed above in this. If you want to develop your eating pattern, that's fine as well; make sure not a lot of carbs are on your plate in your first meal as this will make you binge eat later. Making sure you don't overeat is essential for intermittent fasting, as it will dictate your goals. If you are looking to lose weight, then make sure you eat portion-controlled meals instead of eating whatever your heart desires. These are all the primary tips, make sure you follow them, so you don't end up giving up too soon.

All in all, these tips will help you in the future. As you will see, how much easier fasting becomes for you once you start considering these tips, but don't forget to listen to your body as we previously mentioned. Looking out for your health first is very important, so if you feel like these tips are not helping you within three weeks, then modify your fasting.

Chapter 7: Manage the Symptoms of Menopause

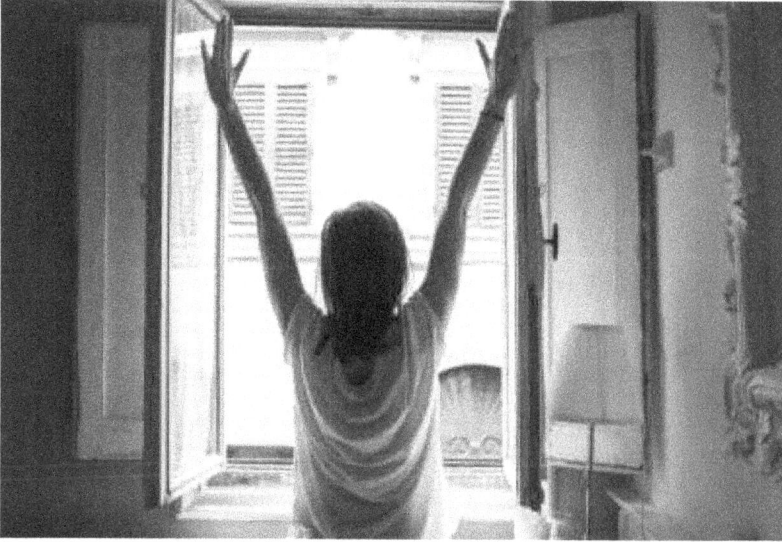

We will discuss all of the issues someone might face when following intermittent fasting, we will also touch upon menopause and how to take care of it appropriately. Intermittent fasting truly is a great way to live the life you want. We will give you all the good and the bad about intermittent fasting, getting you all geared up to get started.

Don't Test the Limits

You must never try to stretch the fasting too far. You have to fast and then give your body the time to recover. If you are beginning fasting, never fast on consecutive days. Always allow your body the time to recover.

Don't Fast Too Long

Initially, you should begin by creating safe gaps between your meals. Eliminate snacks. Then try to stretch the difference between the meals a bit. Always ensure that the highest amount of time spent without food is at the beginning of the fast. It means it is still better to begin fasts early in the evening as you will not feel hungry. Stretching your fast for too long in the morning wouldn't be a very bright idea. In any case, the fasting duration should be anywhere between 12-14 hours only. Several studies have shown that women get much better results with comparatively shorter fasts than men.

No HIIT on Fasting Days

High-intensity interval training is an energy-demanding activity. It should be avoided at all costs on the fasting days, especially if you are beginning your intermittent fasting. It can drain you and create intense energy demands.

No Fasting During the Menstrual Cycle

There is significant blood loss during the periods, and your body needs a lot of rest. Your hormones are also going crazy during this time. Therefore, you must not practice intermittent fasting at this time. Have a Healthy Diet Food choices are critical in the case of women as their nutritional requirements are high.

You must choose a very healthy diet full of all the nutrients so that your hormones remain in check. You should stop fasting if you notice the following things:

• Irregular periods or complete absence of periods

• Sudden resurfacing of sleep disorders without any apparent reason

- On facing sudden and drastic metabolic and digestive issues

- On experiencing sudden mood swings and brain fog

- On having sudden changes in the color of the skin or hair texture

Intermittent Fasting is NOT for you if:

- You have eating disorders

- Have got pregnant or trying to conceive

- Have sleep disorders

- Have adrenal fatigue

- You are suffering from PMS, PCOS, PCOD, Fibroids, Endometriosis, or other hormonal issues

Intermittent fasting isn't a diet. It is a routine. Diets are restrictive; routines are liberating as they flow with life. You always find time to do things while following a method as they are just a part of life. I don't believe people on diets would be able to say the same.

So, you must make it clear in your mind that intermittent fasting isn't a diet. The biggest reason for foods to fail is that they put so many restrictions that people may or may not lose their weight, but they lose their peace of mind. Imagine yourself at a party with people eating and merrymaking. Then imagine yourself standing in one corner sulking as you can't eat anything. Most of the food items that you like are there, but you can't have them.

The steel-clad resolve of sticking to the diet flies out of the window that very moment. The people who can keep the resolve start developing a feeling of resentment. Food is an essential requirement in life. It is needed for satisfying physical, mental, and emotional needs. Anything that is so restrictive cannot be adopted as a lifestyle. Intermittent fasting, on the other hand, is very simple. You only need to remain in the fasted state for a set number of hours in a day or a week.

The kind of diet you want to have, the amount of food you want to eat and the number of hours you want to spend doing an exercise can be up to your own choice. These will all help you in losing weight and staying healthier; however, you would still lose weight even if you don't eat the prescribed food items or don't sweat in the gym for long.

The most significant advantage of intermittent fasting is that it can be quickly adopted as a lifestyle. You don't need to do anything out of the ordinary to follow intermittent fasting. You don't need to prepare elaborate meals. You don't need to be choosy every time you have to decide to eat something. Healthy eating is always advisable, but that doesn't mean you have to get extra picky. Intermittent fasting is a straightforward routine where you will have a certain number of hours in a day to eat. The remaining hours will be the fasting hours, and in them, you can't have anything besides the exempted items listed on the meal plan.

The best thing is that after some time of practicing intermittent fasting, staying hungry for extra-long wouldn't remain a problem at all. It is more about when to eat and less about what or how much to eat Intermittent fasting lays great emphasis on when to eat.

The simple reasons for that are:

• Frequent meals cause significant damage to our system as they keep our gut under constant pressure.

• The blood sugar levels remain consistently high as you keep eating food at short intervals.

• The insulin spike is also there, and hence, you remain prone to insulin sensitivity.

• It also increases cholesterol levels.

• Chronic inflammation also rises.

• Your body is not able to achieve satiety.

• Organs need to work extra hard to adjust the extra energy. All this can be avoided by simply reducing the number of meals in a day. You don't need to reduce the number of calories you have in a day.

You can still have your 2000 calories if you like. You can have even more if you want. You can also eat the pancakes once in a while and again lose weight because your body now has the time to focus on other things besides just digesting food. The human body has passed through a long evolutionary process, and hence, it knows the methods that can help it run smoothly. The recent overexposure to food has complicated things a bit as the body not only gets busy in dealing with the extra energy, but it also has to deal with food items that are not very healthy. Once you start giving it the time to digest the food and begin the necessary processes, it can quickly deal with the kind of food you eat.

Therefore, the real emphasis in intermittent fasting would always remain on maintaining the fasting state for a definite period in a day. We can divide the day into two segments:

The Fasting Window: This is the time of the day during which you can't eat anything at all. There are some exceptions like unsweetened black tea or coffee, unsweetened fresh lime water, or green tea that you can still have in this period as these don't add any calories or don't initiate your digestive process. Besides these items in limited quantity, you need to remain in a completely fasted state during this period. The fasting window is comparatively more prolonged than the eating window. However, you can set the duration of the fasting window as per your convenience and tolerance.

The Eating Window: This is the time of the day during which you can eat. It is always advisable to have a smaller number of meals in a day. You must try to eliminate snacks and unnecessary munching as it leads to cravings and also causes insulin resistance, however, you can eat your fill in your eating windows. There are no calorie caps in intermittent fasting protocols. You need to make your meals as fulfilling as possible so that you don't feel the need to have snacks in between your meals. Healthy food items in the meals are always excellent. They would help you in fighting obesity and chronic inflammation.

However, you can bring these changes one at a time, and there will not be a need to rush the process. The most important part of this to remember will always be to maintain fasting and eating windows.

Things to make everything easy for you.

Exercise and especially, high-intensity interval training, works wonders if you are following intermittent fasting. The reason is simple; intermittent fasting boosts the production of hormones that can increase fat burn. High-intensity interval training creates the right environment at the right time. You may be engaging in high-intensity physical activity later in the day too. But the effects wouldn't be the same as at that time; you would be in a fed state. In that case, there will be no presence of HGH in your bloodstream. This is a hormone which can only be present when you are on an empty stomach after a long fasting interval. It acts as a potent steroid, which is so potent that sports organizations have banned its use as it improves the performance of the athletes.

Therefore, exercise works in intermittent fasting. Not only high-intensity interval training but light cardio exercises, yoga, and aerobics also have their definitive health benefits. If you want to reap the full benefits of intermittent fasting, you must include training in your schedule.

Healthy Food

In this whole book, we have stressed the least on food. It has been intentional so that you can focus entirely on the process and its advantages. However, this doesn't mean that food doesn't play an essential role in fulfilling your objectives, or it isn't crucial. First, healthy food is necessary.

You must try to consume as much fresh and unprocessed food as possible. Staying away from syrups, juices, jam, and jellies is always advisable as these things increase the number of calories consumed but don't give anything to your body. You must always avoid such situations. Still, eat fruits with their pulp. Throwing away the flesh and drinking only the juice is the most significant loss you will face ever. Maintaining a balance among the macronutrients is also very important as reducing the number of meals consumed in a day also affects your calorie intake. If you do not have a balanced diet, you can get nutrient deficient. Therefore, having a healthy diet helps in burning body fat and reducing weight. If your goal is explicitly fat burning, then you should take a keto diet along with intermittent fasting. Keto diet is a high-fat, low-carb diet that helps your body in switching to burning solid fuel in place of glucose fuel. Once that process begins, fat burning becomes very fast and effective. This is simply a suggestion, and you can make do with any healthy eating plan. Recipes will be available for you in this book.

A Positive Attitude

Your attitude plays a vital role whenever bringing any change is considered. With a pessimistic attitude, a person may even lose hope of success or survival is falling even in a small pool. It is not the swimming skills that keep a person afloat but the will and confidence to survive. Recently, a Mexican survived in the Pacific Ocean for 438 days. No amount of swimming skills could have saved a person for that long in the Pacific. However, it was the optimism and will to survive that kept him alive. Weight loss can get disappointing and disheartening at times.

The reaction of people and over conscious attitude at times makes people look for faster results, and they don't follow procedure and then fail. Such things should never be taken to heart. You must always have confidence and the will to succeed. You must keep making adjustments to get the desired results, but looking for shortcuts can lead to failures. Health should always be a long-term goal, as this is the only thing that matters in the end.

Chapter 8: Recipes + 10-Day Plan

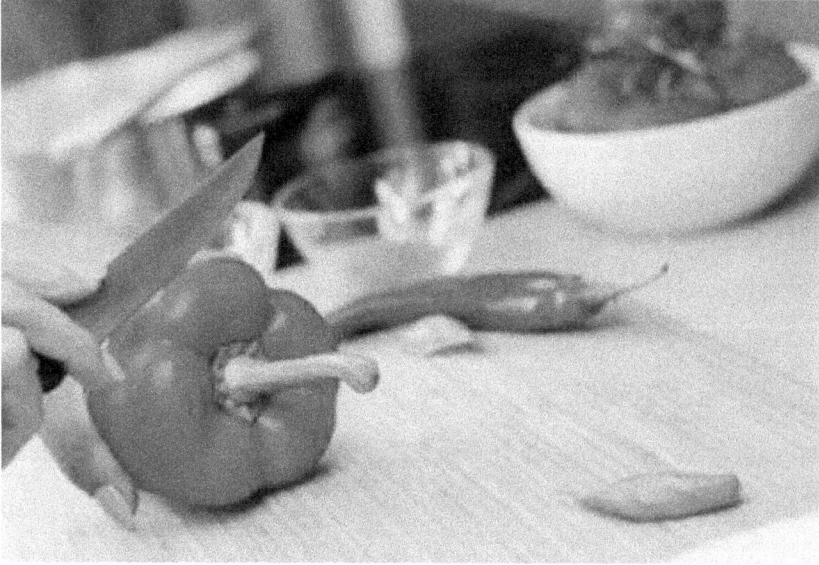

In this chapter, we will be giving you some fantastic low calories recipes, which will not only help you to lose body fat and to put on muscle. These recipes are very low in calories, which will allow you to fill up quite quickly, and they're also nutritionally dense that will also allow you to be more successful in putting on muscle losing fat or whatever it is that you're trying to achieve. The great thing about intermittent fasting is that it is ideal for any goal; the main benefits of intermittent fasting is to detoxify you and to be overall healthy being.

10-Day Plan

Now in this chapter, we will also help you to figure out the right eating plan and give you a 10-day for eating plans that you are in a high position to not only put on muscle or to lose fat butt to make intermittent fasting a habit. This is the main take away from this book, you need to make sure that you make intermittent fasting your practices of a you start seeing the results that you have been looking for Now we will a general example of how you will be eating in a 16/8 fasting protocol, as making a full eating plan could be redundant and pointless, as it is very easy to make the eating plan yourself once you get the idea behind it.

That being said, let's give you the eating plan. This plan is based on your fasting from 6:30 am till 10 am, I know this isn't exactly 16 hours, but half an hour here and there is fine. This protocol will work great for you, in conjunction with the fantastic recipes we have to offer you. The trick with intermittent fasting is to find tasty foods to eat during your fast, so you don't regret it.

Meal 1: 10- 10:30

Breakfast recipes from below

Meal 2: 12 - 12:30

Snack

Meal 3: 3 - 3:30

Lunch recipe from below

Meal 4: 6 - 6:30

Dinner recipes from below

Follow this eating plan for ten days, and you should be in a high position to seeing amazing results and to make this a full-blown habit. The main take away would be to make intermittent fasting an eating habit instead of a diet.

Breakfast

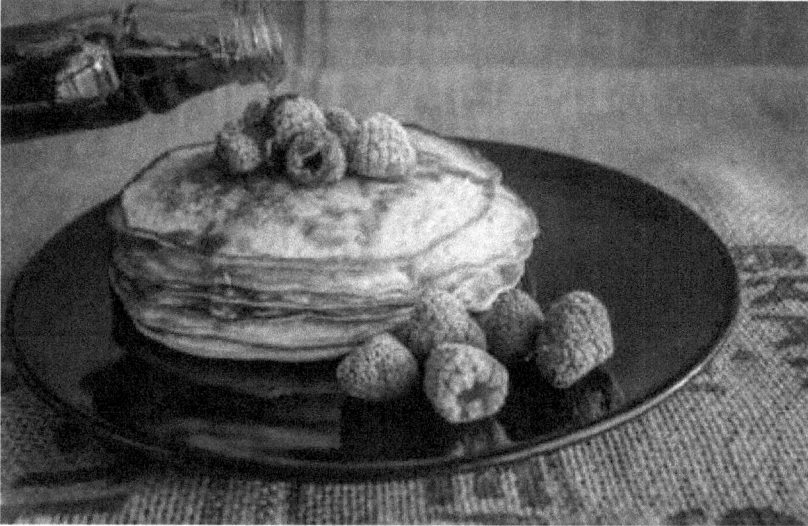

Crustless Broccoli Sun-dried Tomato Quiche

This crustless tofu quiche is low in cholesterol and high in protein. This can be served hot or cold and can be made in muffin tins for an on-the-go breakfast that packs a protein punch.

Ingredients:
12.3-ounce box extra-firm tofu drained and dried

1 ½ cup broccoli, chopped

2 leeks, cleaned and sliced; both white and green parts

2 tablespoons vegetable broth

3 tablespoons nutritional yeast

111

2 chopped cloves of garlic

1 lemon, juiced

2 teaspoons yellow mustard

1 tablespoon tahini

1 tablespoon cornstarch

¼ cup old fashioned oats

½ teaspoon turmeric

3-4 dashes Tabasco sauce

½-1 teaspoon salt

½ cup artichoke hearts, chopped

2/3 cup tomatoes, sun-dried, soaked in hot water

1/8 cup vegetable broth

Instructions:

1. Preheat your oven to 375 degrees Fahrenheit.
2. Prepare a 9" pie plate or springform pan with parchment paper or cooking spray.
3. Put all of the leeks and broccoli on a cookie sheet and drizzle with vegetable broth, salt, and pepper. Bake for about 20-30 min.
4. In the meantime, add the tofu, garlic, nutritional yeast, lemon juice, mustard, tahini, cornstarch, oats, turmeric, salt, and a few dashes of Tabasco in a food processor. When the mixture is smooth, taste for heat and add more Tabasco as needed.

5. Place cooked vegetables with artichoke hearts and tomatoes in a large bowl. With a spatula, scrape in tofu mixture from the processor. Mix carefully, so all of the vegetables are well distributed. If the mixture seems too dry, add a little vegetable broth or water.
6. Add mixture to pie plate muffin tins, or springform pan and spread evenly.
7. Bake for about 35 min. or until lightly browned.
8. Cool before serving. It is delicious, both warm and chilled!

Chocolate Pancakes

Everyone deserves chocolate for breakfast every once in a while. Satisfy your sweet tooth with these gluten-free, vegan chocolate pancakes that go well with almost any fruit of choice, especially strawberries, bananas, and raspberries.

Ingredients:

1 ¼ cup gluten-free flour of choice

1 tablespoon ground flaxseed

1 tablespoon baking powder

3 tablespoons nutritional yeast

2 tablespoons unsweetened cocoa powder

¼ teaspoon of sea salt

1 cup unsweetened, unflavored almond milk

1 tablespoon vegan mini chocolate chips (optional)

1 teaspoon vanilla extract

¼ teaspoon stevia powder or 1 tablespoon pure maple syrup

1 tablespoon apple cider vinegar

¼ cup unsweetened applesauce.

Instructions:

1. Get a medium bowl and mix all the dry ingredients (flour, baking powder, flaxseed, cocoa powder, yeast, salt, and optional chocolate chips). Whisk until evenly combined.

2. In a separate small bowl, combine wet ingredients except for the applesauce (almond milk, vanilla extract, apple cider vinegar, maple syrup, or stevia powder).

3. Add wet ingredient mixture and applesauce to the dry ingredients and mix by hand until ingredients are just combined.

4. The batter should sit for 10 minutes. It will rise and thicken, possibly doubling in size.

5. Heat an electric griddle or nonstick skillet to medium heat and spray with a small amount of nonstick spray, if desired. Scoop batter into 3-inch rounds. Much like traditional pancakes, bubbles will start to appear. When bubbles start to burst, flip pancakes and cook for 1-2 minutes. Yields 12 pancakes.

Breakfast Scramble

Here is another egg-free breakfast option for the veggie lover! Many scramble recipes call for tofu, whereas here we are using cauliflower. This recipe is versatile and allows you to use whichever veggies you may already have in your refrigerator. Feel free to substitute at will!

Ingredients:
1 large head cauliflower, cut up

1 seeded, diced green bell pepper

1 seeded, diced red bell pepper

2 cups sliced mushrooms (approximately 8 oz whole mushrooms)

1 peeled, diced red onion

3 peeled, minced cloves of garlic

Sea salt

1 ½ teaspoons turmeric

1–2 tablespoons of low-sodium soy sauce

¼ cup nutritional yeast (optional)

½ teaspoon black pepper

Instructions:

1. Sauté green and red peppers, mushrooms, and onion in a medium saucepan or skillet over medium-high heat until onion is translucent (should be 7–8 min). Add an occasional

tablespoon or two of water to the pan to prevent vegetables from sticking.

2. Add cauliflower and cook until florets are tenders. It should be 5 to 6 minutes.

3. Add, pepper, garlic, soy sauce, turmeric, and yeast (if using) to the pan and cook for about 5 minutes.

Superfood Breakfast Bars

Need a quick pre-made breakfast option you can grab and go? This breakfast bar is not only sweet and salty, but it's also vegan, gluten-free, and packed with superfood energy.

Ingredients:

4 apples

1.5 cups mix of mulberries and goji berries, soaked in lukewarm water for about 30 minutes

1 cup all-natural apple juice + 3 tablespoons divided

2 tablespoons maple syrup

2-3 tablespoons sunflower seed butter

2 teaspoons aluminum-free baking powder

4 cups gluten-free certified oats

Pinch of cinnamon (optional)

Sunflower seeds for garnish

Instructions:

1. Preheat your oven to 390 degrees Fahrenheit.

2. Line the 11" x 8" baking dish with parchment paper.

3. Chop apples coarsely and remove seeds. Add to blender with 1 c. of the apple juice. Blend until smooth

4. Mix the remaining 3 tablespoons of apple juice, sunflower butter, and maple syrup in a small bowl. You will create a creamy and smooth paste.

5. In a large bowl, combine the soaked and trained berries, oats, sunflower paste, baking powder, and apple mix into a well-mixed dough.

6. Press the dough with a spatula or your hands in the baking dish. Top it with sunflower seeds. Bake for 20 min.

Lunch

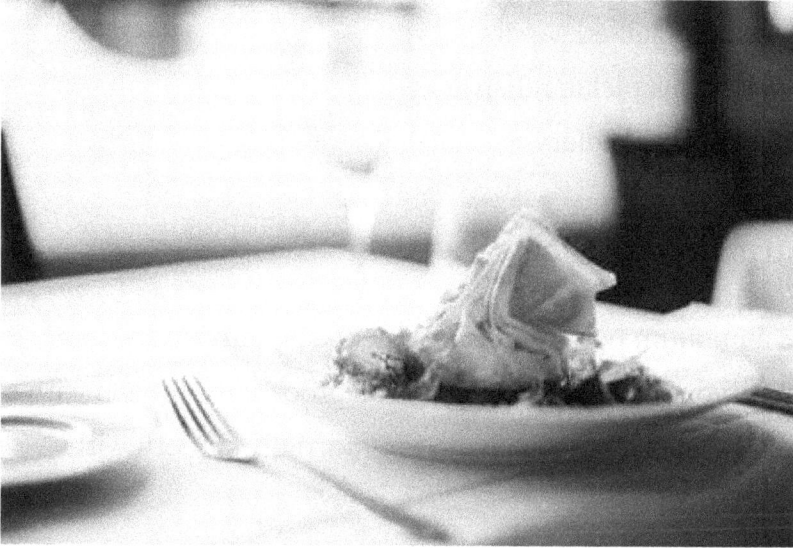

Vegan Tuna Salad

This "tuna salad" recipe includes inexpensive, easy to find ingredients that can be made in advance and stored in the refrigerator for about a week. Serve on a bed of greens, your favorite crackers, or as a classic sandwich. Feel free to add ingredients for flavor and texture, such as carrots or bell peppers.

Ingredients:

2 cans chickpeas

1 tablespoon prepared yellow mustard

2 tablespoons vegan mayonnaise

1 tablespoon jarred capers

2 tablespoons pickle relish

½ cup chopped celery

Instructions:

1. In a medium bowl, combine chickpeas, mustard, vegan mayo, and mustard. Pulse in a food processor or mash with a potato masher until the mixture is partially smooth with some chunks.

2. Add the remaining ingredients to the chickpea mixture and mix until combined.

3. Serve immediately or refrigerate until ready to serve.

Veggie Wrap with Apples and Spicy Hummus

Wraps are a versatile and portable lunch option that can be adapted to any taste. The combination of the soft hummus and broccoli slaw creates a balanced texture of smoothness and crunchiness. The spicy hummus with apple brings a unique sweet and spicy blend. The end result: a lunch wrap that is anything but boring.

Ingredients:

1 tortilla of your choice: flour, corn, gluten-free, etc.

3-4 tablespoons of your favorite spicy hummus (a plain hummus mixed with salsa is good, too!)

A few leaves of your favorite leafy greens

¼ apple sliced thin

½ cup broccoli slaw (store-bought or homemade are both goods)

½ teaspoon lemon juice

2 teaspoons dairy-free, plain, unsweetened yogurt

Salt and pepper to taste

Instructions:

1. Mix broccoli slaw with lemon juice and yogurt. Add pepper and salt to taste and mix well.

2. Lay tortilla flat.

3. Spread hummus all over the tortilla.

4. Lay down leafy greens on hummus.

5. On one half, pile broccoli slaw over lettuce. Place apples on top of the slaw.

6. Starting with the half with slaw and apples, roll tortilla tightly.

7. Cut in half if desired and enjoy!

Mac and Cheese Bites

Welcome to the vegan twist on an old classic. We promised this book would help satisfy some of your old, pre-vegan cravings, so here's a great portable comfort food bite that will satisfy kids and grown-ups alike. Note that these can be eaten warm or cool, though warming them up may make them fall apart a bit.

Ingredients:

1 ½ cups uncooked macaroni (gluten-free will work if needed)

1 medium onion, chopped (can substitute with 1 medium yellow pepper if you don't care for onions.)

1 clove garlic, chopped

2 tablespoons cornstarch, or arrowroot powder

1 cup non-dairy milk

½ teaspoon smoked paprika (can substitute for chipotle powder)

1 teaspoon lemon juice or apple cider vinegar

½ cup nutritional yeast

1 teaspoon salt

Instructions:

1. Preheat your oven to 350 degrees Fahrenheit.

2. Prepare the muffin tin with liners.

3. Prepare macaroni according to instructions.

4. While macaroni is cooking, sauté garlic and onion (or substitute of choice) until it is just starting to turn golden brown. This can be done in a dry pan, but adding some oil will work as well.

5. Add garlic, onion, and all other non-macaroni ingredients into a blender and mix until smooth.

6. Drain the macaroni and return to the pan.

7. Pour sauce over macaroni and stir well.

8. Spoon mixture into muffin tin, stirring occasionally in between such an equal amount of sauce goes in each cup.

9. Push down tops with the back of a spoon.

10. Bake in the oven for 30 min.

11. Serve once cooled.

Chick'n Salad with Cranberries and Pistachios

This recipe calls for soy curls (or textured vegetable protein) for the "chick'n," but you could easily use tempeh or another meat substitute for choice. This salad can be served on a bed of greens, put into a wrap, or on bread as a traditional sandwich.

Ingredients:

1 ½ cups dry soy curls (textured vegetable protein)

2 dashes apple cider vinegar

½ cup diced granny smith apples (approx. 1 small apple)

¼ cup shelled pistachios, chopped

½ cup dried cranberries

5-6 tablespoons veganaise (adjust depending on how creamy you would like the salad to be)

1 teaspoon of sea salt

A pinch of thyme

Instructions:

1. Soak soy curls in warm water for 10 min. Squeeze excess water out of them and roughly chop larger pieces. Set aside.

2. While soy curls are soaking, mix diced apple and vinegar. Drain any excess liquid.

3. Combine apples with all other ingredients in large bowl until ingredients are evenly mixed. Add seasoning to taste. Chill for at least 30 minutes. Serve as desired.

Dinner

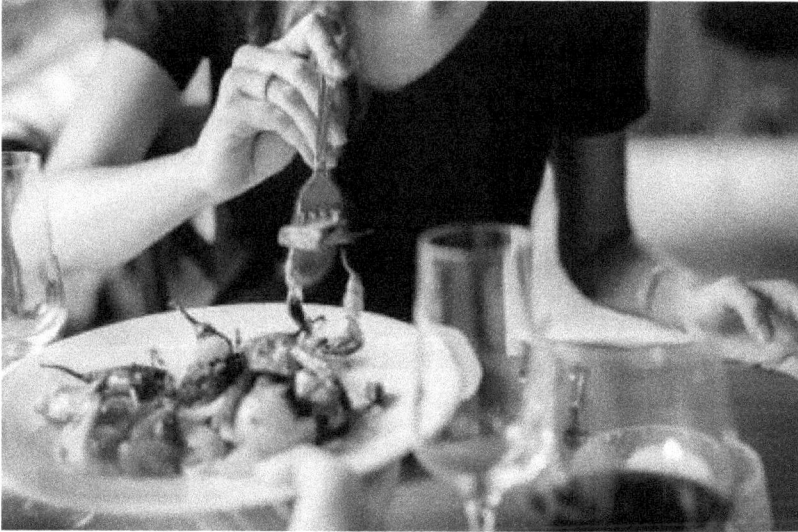

End the day with these satisfying, belly-filling dinners that are great for families and solo homes alike.

Pan-fried Jackfruit over Pasta with Lemon Coconut Cream Sauce

This creamy, lemony coconut sauce can be served with a variety of meat alternatives. Jackfruit gives the dish a hint of sweetness to break through the richness of the cream sauce.

Ingredients:

1 lb. pasta of choice

2 cans jackfruit in brine

2 tablespoons flour of choice

Garlic powder, dried oregano, paprika, black pepper, kosher salt to taste

2 tablespoons vegetable oil

4 tablespoons vegan butter

2 cups of coconut milk

Juice of 1 lemon

2 tablespoons grated vegan parmesan cheese

1 pinch ground nutmeg

1 teaspoon lemon zest (can use the same lemon from juice)

Fresh basil leaves, chopped for garnish

Instructions:

1. Cook pasta until al dente. Drain the pasta but reserve 1 cup of the pasta water. Set it aside for now.

2. While the pasta is cooking, drain the jackfruit and cut each piece in half. Pat jackfruit dry.

3. Mix flour with garlic powder, oregano, paprika, pepper, and salt in a separate bowl.

4. Toss flour mixture with jackfruit.

5. Heat vegetable oil in a skillet. Pan-fry the jackfruit until crisp on both sides. It takes around ten minutes in total.

6. Transfer the jackfruit to a plate lined with a paper towel and set aside.

7. In a large saucepan or skillet, melt vegan butter. Add coconut milk and lemon juice. Then add parmesan cheese and nutmeg. Cook until sauce is thick.

8. Add cooked pasta and half of the reserved pasta water to skillet. Toss to coat all pasta.

9. Cook until everything is hot and the sauce is to desired consistency and pasta is heated through. If the sauce is too thick, continue to use remaining pasta water.

10. Turn off heat. Add lemon zest and add pepper and salt to taste. Sprinkle parmesan and basil leaves. Add pan-fried jackfruit on top when serving.

Butternut Squash Tacos with Tempeh Chorizo

This dish comes together quite easily, though there are a few preparation tips recommended you do in advance. If you have challenges with digesting beans or soy, steam your tempeh before using it. Simmer the butternut squash in veggie broth or water and vinegar as this adds more flavor in lieu of steaming. Keep a little extra water on hand in case the squash starts to stick.

Ingredients:

One 8-ounce package tempeh

½ cup of filtered water

¼ cup apple cider vinegar

2 cups butternut squash, peeled, cut into cubes

1 teaspoon chili powder

½ teaspoon smoked paprika

½ teaspoon cumin

½ teaspoon garlic powder

½ teaspoon oregano

A dash of cayenne

1 tablespoon nutritional yeast

A few dashes of liquid smoke

Black pepper and sea salt to taste

½ cup thinly julienned carrot (optional)

8 corn tortillas (or whatever you have on hand)

1 large avocado, pitted and sliced

Cilantro, chopped

Instructions:

1. Cut the tempeh into two parts. Steam for 10 min. Place in a large bowl and tear apart into small pieces either with your hands (after it's cooled) or with a pastry cutter.

2. While tempeh is steaming, bring water and vinegar to a boil in a small skillet.

3. Add spices, squash, liquid smoke, nutritional yeast, and a pinch of sea salt to skillet. Coat well and simmer covered, stirring occasionally. Add carrots and tempeh, covering again. Simmer a little while longer, stirring to prevent sticking. Uncover and season with pepper and salt.

4. Fill warmed tortillas with squash and tempeh mix and top with avocado and cilantro.

Vegan Fish Sticks and Tartar Sauce

This recipe for the so-called "wish" sticks as some call it. This has been kid-tested and approved, though adults can enjoy them on a sandwich or a salad topper.

Ingredients:

Fish Sticks:

12-ounce package extra-firm tofu

½ cup cornmeal

1 tablespoon garlic powder

1 tablespoon dried basil

2 tablespoons dulse flakes

1 tablespoon onion powder

½ cup whole wheat flour (rice flour is a good gluten-free option)

10 turns fresh black pepper

1 tablespoon of sea salt

¼ cup non-dairy milk, unsweetened

1 cup high-heat oil for frying

Vegan Tartar Sauce:

¼ cup sweet pickle relish

½ cup vegan mayo

½ teaspoon sugar

½ teaspoon lemon juice

5 turns fresh black pepper

Instructions:

1. Rinse tofu and drain in a colander. Placing a heavy plate on tofu with a heavy item on top will help drain better. Set it aside.

2. In a medium bowl, mix the flour, cornmeal, garlic powder, basil, onion powder, dulse flakes, pepper, and salt. Whisk together. Set the mix aside.

3. Set tofu on cutting board. Cut into quarters.

4. Slice tofu into thin pieces. You should have 28-32 pieces in total.

5. In a large cast-iron skillet, heat oil on medium/low heat.

6. In a small bowl, pour non-dairy milk.

7. Dip each piece of tofu in non-dairy milk. Immediately dip in breading, coating all sides evenly. Repeat until all pieces are coated.

8. The oil will start to splatter when hot enough. At that point, add tofu pieces to skillet. Repeat until all pieces are cooked.

9. Each side will cook for about 2-3 minutes. Watch for golden brown color. Place tofu pieces on a brown paper bag as you remove them from pan to soak up excess oil.

10. Repeat as necessary until all tofu is cooked. Cool before serving. Mix all tartar sauce ingredients until an even and creamy sauce is made. Enjoy!

Vegan Philly Cheesesteak

A great twist on a regional favorite, this sandwich is fairly simple to put together and contains ingredients that are easy to find. It can be served with vegan mayo if desired.

Ingredients:

6-8 sliced Portobello mushrooms

4 cloves garlic, minced

1 tablespoon olive oil

1 whole clove garlic

½ teaspoon black pepper

1 teaspoon dried thyme

½ large diced onion

A dash of kosher salt

1 tablespoon vegan Worcestershire sauce

Hoagie rolls or another small loaf of bread of choice

1 cup shredded vegan cheddar cheese

Vegan mayo (optional)

Instructions:

1. Preheat the broiler.

2. In a deep skillet, heat olive oil. Brown mushrooms in oil, about 10 min.

3. Add thyme, garlic, and pepper until evenly coated.

4. Add onion and salt. Mushrooms must be well cooked before adding salt. Cook until onion is caramelized and softened, which should be for about 5 minutes. Add Worcestershire sauce and mix well.

5. Slice the bread lengthwise. Coat open sides of bread with olive oil or cooking spray. To add garlic flavor, cut the whole garlic clove, cut off the tip, and put on the oiled side of bread. Garlic powder is also a good substitute.

6. If desired, add optional vegan mayo. Place bread on cookie sheet. Fill loaves with mushrooms and top with shredded vegan cheddar cheese.

7. Place in broiler until cheese has melted, which should be 4-5 minutes.

Desserts and Snacks

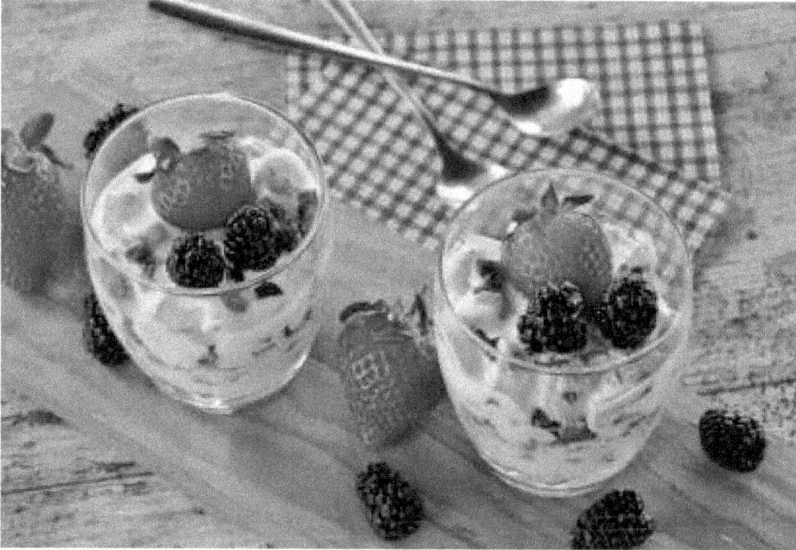

Switching to a refined sugar-free, plant-based lifestyle doesn't have to mean depriving yourself of your sweet tooth cravings. Make these for your own late-night treat or multiply the ingredients for family gatherings.

Mango Lime Chia Pudding

Chia pudding is another versatile treat that can be used at breakfast or as a mid-day snack. Pack it in a mason jar or a recycled food jar. This is one of many flavor combinations you can create.

Ingredients:

3 cups fresh or frozen mango chunks

One 15.5-ounce can coconut milk

1 tablespoon lime zest

¼ cup maple syrup

¼ cup freshly squeezed lime juice

¼ cup hemp seeds

1/3 cup chia seeds

Topping options: Approximately 8 cups of any combination of mango, banana, pineapple, or any fruit you'd love with mango and lime. (Banana is a fruit you'd want to wait to add until you are ready to eat the pudding as it browns and gets mushy very quickly once out of its peel)

Instructions:

1. Place mango chunks, coconut milk, lime zest, and maple syrup in a blender. Mix until smooth.

2. Add hemp and chia seeds in the blender and stir by hand or blend on low to just combine.

3. This should yield 4 cups of pudding. Portion it as you prefer. One suggestion is to divide into 8 portions, one each in a pint jar, and top with one cup of fresh fruit.

4. Refrigerate pudding until ready to eat, minimum 4 hours to set. The pudding keeps for 5-7 days.

Mint Chocolate Truffle Larabar Bites

This copycat recipe can be rolled into individual balls or placed in a pan and cut up as bars after firming in the refrigerator. With 15-minute prep time, this quick fix will satisfy any sweet tooth! Can keep for 3 weeks if refrigerated in an airtight container.

Ingredients:

1 cup vegan chocolate chips (semi-sweet dark chips are recommended)

10 large Medjool dates

1 ½ cups of raw almonds

¼ cup coconut flour

¼ cup of cocoa powder

¼-1/2 teaspoon peppermint extract

2 tablespoons water

Instructions:

1. Pour almonds into a food processor and chop until a fine flour.

2. Add chocolate chips, dates, flour and cocoa, and process again until well combined.

3. Add oil and peppermint extract.

4. Process one more time until the mix starts balling up.

5. Taste a small bit and add more peppermint if you wish. Process again if you do.

6. Remove the blade from the processor and form the dough into balls. Choose whatever size you like, as they do not need to bake and will be good in any portion.

Peanut Butter Caramel Rice Krispies

Take a trip down memory lane and bring the wonderful memory of rice Krispie treats into the adult world. This healthier version will give you a light and crunchy snack that is great for munching at home or family potlucks.

Ingredients:

6 cups crisp rice cereal

1/3 cup creamy peanut butter (can substitute with almond or sunflower seed butter)

¾ cup brown rice syrup

1 teaspoon vanilla extract

¼ cup maple syrup

Peanut butter drizzle:

2 tablespoons creamy peanut butter (or substitute of choice)

1 teaspoon maple syrup (or another liquid sweetener)

1-2 teaspoons to thin, if needed

Instructions:

1. Line a 9" x 9" square pan with parchment or wax paper. An 8" x 8" pan will work as well. Treats will just be thicker.

2. Place a large pot over medium heat. Add brown rice syrup and maple syrup in and bring it to a rolling boil. Cook for 1-2 minutes, stirring often and making sure mix does not burn.

144

3. Remove from heat. Mix in vanilla and peanut butter with whisk until smooth.

4. In a large bowl, pour in crisp rice cereal. Stir in the liquid mix until well combined.

5. Scoop into pan and spread out evenly. Press down with wet fingers or spatula. Place in freezer to set for 10 minutes while making peanut butter drizzle.

6. In a separate microwavable bowl, mix together peanut butter and maple syrup. Microwave in 30-second intervals until just warm for easier mixing. Add 1 teaspoon water at a time if needed. Mix until smooth.

7. Remove treats from the freezer and drizzle on the peanut butter mix. Place back in the freezer until firm, about 10 min.

8. Cut into squares for serving. Bars will hold their shape quite well at room temperature but can be stored in the fridge. Leftovers can be wrapped up and kept in the fridge for 5 to 7 days or freeze for up to one month.

Easy Chocolate Pudding

Get ready to throw away the instant boxed stuff and try this equally easy, dairy-free chocolate pudding that is so rich, creamy, and chocolatey that you won't believe that it's healthy and refined sugar-free. Top with coconut whipped cream for a perfect treat.

Ingredients:

1 ½ cups organic coconut cream from a can

½ cup raw cacao powder (sifted unsweetened cocoa powder works as well)

6 tablespoons pure maple syrup (may adjust to up to 8 tablespoons, depending on how sweet you like it)

2 teaspoons pure vanilla extract

Fine-grain sea salt

Instructions:

1. In a small saucepan over low heat, whisk coconut cream, cacao, and maple syrup until smooth. A smaller whisk my make a smoother mixture. Continue to cook over low/medium for 2 minutes, or until the mixture just starts to come to a boil with small bubbles.

2. Remove from heat. Add salt and vanilla. Stir. Taste and add more maple if you'd like a sweeter pudding.

3. Pour into individual containers/bowls or keep in one larger bowl to set.

4. Cover and refrigerate until set, or overnight for a thick and creamy pudding. Makes 4 servings.

Conclusion

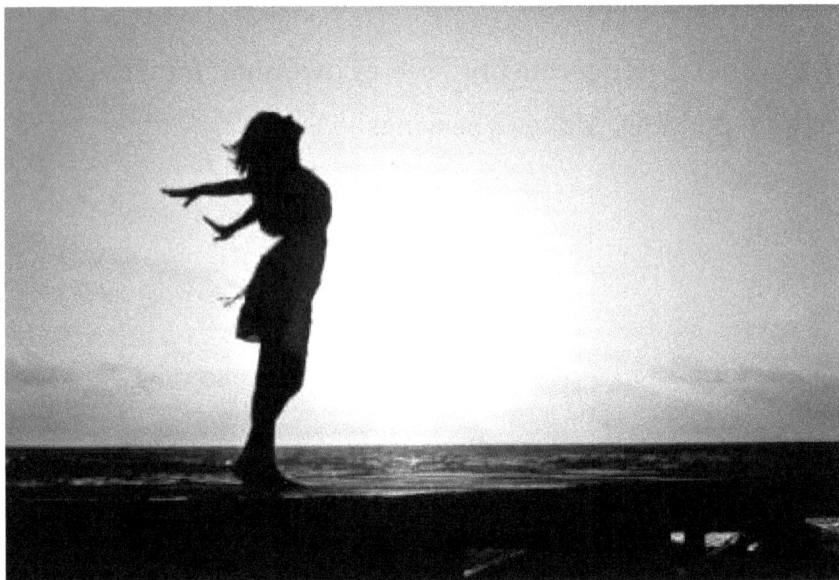

Thank you so much for reading this book, *Intermittent Fasting Over 50: The Ultimate and Complete Guide for Healthy Weight Loss, Burn Fat, Slow Aging, Detox Your Body, and Support Your Hormones with the Process of Metabolic Autophagy,* till the end. Now the best thing for you to do would be to start implementing all the information provided to you in this book. Intermittent fasting will truly change your life for the better. Please don't just read this book and not do anything about it.

We have given you a full proof plan, with recipes and eating schedule. You should have no problem executing it, now go ahead and start bettering your health.

www.ingramcontent.com/pod-product-compliance
Lightning Source LLC
Chambersburg PA
CBHW050730030426
42336CB00012B/1500